Spatial Analysis in Epidemiology

Spatial Analysis in Epidemiology

Dirk U. Pfeiffer
Epidemiology Division, Royal Veterinary College, University of London,
United Kingdom

Timothy P. Robinson
Food and Agricultural Organization of the United Nations, Italy

Mark Stevenson
Epicentre, Institute of Veterinary, Animal and Biomedical Sciences,
Massey University, New Zealand

Kim B. Stevens
Epidemiology Division, Royal Veterinary College, University of London,
United Kingdom

David J. Rogers
Department of Zoology, Oxford University, United Kingdom

Archie C. A. Clements
Division of Epidemiology and Social Medicine, School of Population
Health, University of Queensland, Australia

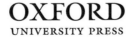

OXFORD
UNIVERSITY PRESS

OXFORD

UNIVERSITY PRESS

Great Clarendon Street, Oxford OX2 6DP

Oxford University Press is a department of the University of Oxford.
It furthers the University's objective of excellence in research, scholarship,
and education by publishing worldwide in

Oxford New York

Auckland Cape Town Dar es Salaam Hong Kong Karachi
Kuala Lumpur Madrid Melbourne Mexico City Nairobi
New Delhi Shanghai Taipei Toronto

With offices in

Argentina Austria Brazil Chile Czech Republic France Greece
Guatemala Hungary Italy Japan Poland Portugal Singapore
South Korea Switzerland Thailand Turkey Ukraine Vietnam

Oxford is a registered trade mark of Oxford University Press
in the UK and in certain other countries

Published in the United States
by Oxford University Press Inc., New York

First published 2008

Reprinted 2009, 2010 (twice)

British Library Cataloguing in Publication Data
Data available

Library of Congress Cataloging in Publication Data
Data available

Typeset by Newgen Imaging Systems (P) Ltd., Chennai, India
Printed in Great Britain
on acid-free paper by
CPI Antony Rowe, Chippenham

ISBN 978-0-19-850988-2 (Hbk.)   978-0-19-850989-9 (Pbk.)

10 9 8 7 6 5 4

Contents

Abbreviations

AIC	Akaike information criterion
ASF	African swine fever
AVHRR	Advanced Very High Resolution Radiometer
AUC	Area under the curve
BPA	Basic probability assignments
BSE	Bovine spongiform encephalopathy
CAR	Conditional autoregressive
CEPP	Cluster Evaluation Permutation Procedure
CJD	Creutzfeldt-Jakob disease
CUSUM	Cumulative sum
DEMP	Density equalized map projection
DBMS	Database management system
DST	Dempster–Shafer theory
EET	Excess events test
EMM	Ederer–Myers–Mantel
ESDA	Exploratory spatial data analysis
FAO	Food and Agriculture Organization of the United Nations
FMD	Foot-and-mouth disease
GAM	Geographical Analysis Machine
GIS	Geographic information systems
GPS	Global positioning system
HEPP	Heterogeneous Poisson process
HGE	Human granulocytic ehrlichiosis
ICC	Intraclass correlation coefficient
IDW	Inverse distance weighting
K-L	Kullback–Leibler
LISA	Local indicators of spatial association
MA	Moving average
MAUP	Modifiable areal unit problem
MCDA	Multicriteria decision analysis
MCDM	Multicriteria decision making
MCMC	Markov chain Monte Carlo
MEET	Maximized excess events test
MLR	Maximum likelihood ratio
NDVI	Normalized Difference Vegetation Index
NNA	Nearest neighbour areas
NOAA	National Oceanic and Atmospheric Administration
ODBC	Open database connectivity

OWA	Ordered weighted averaging
Pmax	Poisson maximum
SAM	Statistical Analysis module
ROC	Receiver operating characteristic
SAR	Simultaneous autoregressive
SARS	Severe acute respiratory syndrome
SD	Standard deviation
SIDS	Sudden infant death syndrome
SIR	Susceptible-infected-recovered
SLE	Systemic lupus erythematosus
SMR	Standardized mortality/morbidity ratio
SQL	Structured Query Language
TB	Tuberculosis
TIN	Triangulated irregular network
UMP	Uniformly most powerful
URISA	Urban and Regional Information Systems Association
VPD	Vapour pressure deficit
WLC	Weighted linear combination

Preface

Over the last 20 years, the application of spatial analysis in the context of epidemiological surveillance and research has increased in an exponential fashion. Having been involved in this field since 1988, first as researchers and then also as postgraduate teachers, we felt there was a need for a textbook that helps to guide epidemiologists and other biologists logically through the complexities of spatial analysis.

This book aims to provide a practical introduction to spatial analysis, by focusing on application rather than theory, and by drawing on a wide range of examples from both human and animal health, including vector-borne and infectious diseases and non-infectious conditions. We provide worked examples of the principal methodologies, using mainly the same disease dataset throughout, which allows for direct comparison of the various techniques and helps to demonstrate their comparative strengths and weaknesses.

The book is written primarily for postgraduate students and postdoctoral researchers embarking upon epidemiological studies that may require the use of spatial analytical methods. However, the methods described are also relevant to students and researchers dealing with spatial data in the fields of ecology, zoology, parasitology, environmental science, geography, and statistics. Whilst the book is written in plain language, avoiding jargon as much as possible, a basic understanding of epidemiology and statistics is assumed.

The sequence around which we have structured the book involves firstly visualizing spatial patterns in data, then describing these spatial patterns, and finally attempting to explain the observed patterns. This further enables us to predict changes in patterns and to use our explanations and predictions to inform decisions and to guide policy formulation. Following an introductory chapter, Chapters 2 and 3 address spatial data and the different ways in which they can be observed and presented. Chapters 4, 5, and 6 elaborate on the methods used to describe and quantify spatial patterns, while Chapter 7 looks at some of the methods that can be used to help explain spatial patterns, mostly in terms of environmental variables. Finally, Chapter 8 looks into ways of assessing disease risk and informing decision-making.

We have tried to be consistent with notation, but where this would lead to clumsiness have not forced ourselves to be so. Where notations deviate from the norm, the context should make this clear. At the risk of becoming fairly quickly outdated, we have included references to specific software programmes and provided links to websites. Whilst these all worked at the time of publishing we cannot guarantee their future validity.

The majority of worked examples presented in the book are based on data collected as part of Great Britain's national bovine tuberculosis (TB) control programme. A subset of the national database, comprising cattle TB data from the period 1986 to 1999 was used with permission from the United Kingdom Department for Environment, Food and Rural Affairs (DEFRA) and was kindly provided by Mr. Andy Mitchell and Dr. Richard Clifton-Hadley of the Veterinary Laboratories Agency (VLA).

The Animal Production and Health Division of the Food and Agriculture Organization of the United Nations (FAO) has supported this work as part of its mandate to build national and international capacity for the formulation of evidence-based disease control policies and strategies. In co-publishing the book, FAO hopes to promote its use among member countries.

The motivation to write this book came from our experience with epidemiological spatial analysis as researchers, as teachers, and as practitioners in policy formulation and advice.

Over the years, we have published numerous reviews on spatial analysis and geographic information systems (GIS) in epidemiology (Sanson et al. 1991; Pfeiffer and Morris 1994; Pfeiffer 2000; Robinson 2000; Pfeiffer and Hugh-Jones 2002; Pfeiffer 2004), have run short courses and distance learning modules in spatial analysis, and have taught spatial analysis as part of the masters' courses at the Royal Veterinary College and the London School of Hygiene and Tropical Medicine.

Through discussions with colleagues and postgraduate students in spatial analysis, it became clear to us that there is no spatial epidemiology textbook that provides a comprehensive introduction to the subject area, yet at the same time is accessible to the wider group of epidemiologists, covering issues from spatial data management to analytical decision support tools. We hope that this book will go at least some of the way towards redressing this shortfall.

We were very fortunate in being able to convince our co-authors Mark Stevenson, Kim Stevens, David Rogers, and Archie Clements to join us in this endeavour. Particular thanks are due to Kim Stevens who, apart from contributing her own material to the book, also took over the editing: without her we would not have been able to complete it.

Dirk U. Pfeiffer
Royal Veterinary College
University of London

Timothy P. Robinson
Food and Agriculture Organization
of the United Nations

CHAPTER 1

Introduction

The transmission of infectious diseases is closely linked to the concepts of spatial and spatio-temporal proximity, as transmission is more likely to occur if the at-risk individuals are close in a spatial and a temporal sense. In the case of non-communicable disease occurrence, proximity to environmental risk factors may be important. Epidemiological analyses therefore have to take both space and time into account, with the basic principle being to examine the dependence amongst observations in relation to these two dimensions. While this appears to be a simple and logical step it introduces a complication, as the inferences resulting from classical statistical analysis methods assume that observations are independent from each other. The consequence of ignoring dependence, if present, is that estimated confidence intervals are narrower than they should be (assuming we are dealing with positive autocorrelation). Consequently, the distinguishing feature of spatial or spatio-temporal statistical methods is that they take account of the spatial or spatio-temporal arrangement (i.e. that observations in space or time are not independent of each other).

Epidemiology is about the quest for knowledge in relation to disease causation, and this can be about understanding risk factors or about the effects of interventions. To demonstrate cause and effect relationships, the philosopher Karl Popper emphasized the need to develop a theoretical hypothesis based on the observed data, which is then converted into a testable hypothesis that can be challenged experimentally. The aim is then to refute or corroborate the testable hypothesis by repeated experimental challenge (Chalmers 1999). Spatial epidemiology is particularly strong in the first part of the Popperian approach to scientific

investigation, but less so when it comes to testing hypotheses through experimentation. The most basic approach is to examine maps of disease occurrence visually, together with data from other map layers, for the purpose of formulating theoretical hypotheses. This mode of investigation, which has also been called the 'gee whiz' effect, suffers from some inherent weaknesses in that it does not involve statistical testing or falsification (Jacquez 1998). Consistent with Popper's philosophy, it needs to be followed by statistical assessment and experimental challenge of the hypotheses before inferences in relation to cause and effect can be drawn. Spatial epidemiology provides the necessary tools for such statistical assessment, although many of these tools are still relatively unfamiliar to most epidemiologists. In response to an increased awareness of environmental health hazards, various protocols have been developed to enhance the scientific rigour of investigations aimed at identifying spatial clusters of disease[1]. It does however need to be emphasized that, consistent with all epidemiological investigations, definitive causal inference is difficult, if not impossible, to obtain through analysis of epidemiological data (Jacquez 2004).

Since John Snow's cholera-outbreak investigation in 1854, epidemiology has played an increasingly important role in providing scientific evidence to support animal and human health-policy development (Stolley and Lasky 1995). The assessment of the spatial pattern of the cholera cases in relation to potential risk factors, in this instance the locations of water pumps, was important in identifying the source of the infection (see Fig. 1.1), although

---

[1] http://www.eurocat.ulster.ac.uk/clusterinvprot.html

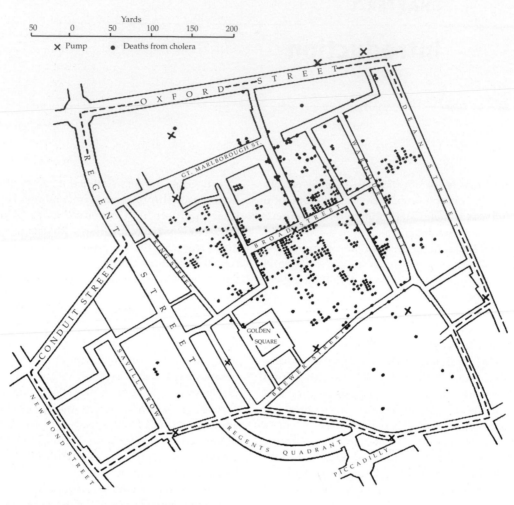

Figure 1.1 John Snow's 1854 cholera-outbreak map of London (deaths shown as dots, water pumps as crosses). Reproduced from Gilbert (1958) with permission from *Blackwell Publishing*.

it is now recognized that the map was probably not the key factor for this cause-effect inference (McLeod 2000).

One of the challenges of the current century is to improve the public's understanding and perception of the value of science, thereby facilitating the more widespread use of health policies that take effective account of up-to-date scientific evidence. Risk communication is an essential element in this process, with the objective being to present scientific outputs in ways that are understandable to non-scientists (Leiss and Powell 2004). One of the mechanisms for improving the transparency and widespread understanding of scientific evidence

is to use visual methods of presentation in order to make fairly abstract quantitative results easier to comprehend, which is where maps can be particularly useful (Bell et al. 2006).

1.1 Framework for spatial analysis

The field of spatial epidemiology includes a wide range of techniques and deciding which ones to use can be challenging. Fig. 1.2 is a diagrammatic representation of a spatial analysis framework adapted from Bailey and Gatrell (1995). The objectives of spatial epidemiological analysis are the description of spatial patterns, identification of disease clusters, and explanation or prediction of disease risk. Fundamental to these objectives is the need for data which, in addition to the classical data attribute information describing the characteristics of the entity studied, require the availability of georeferenced feature data, be they points or areas.

Management of the data is performed using geographic information systems (GIS) and database management systems (DBMS), and is of relevance throughout the various phases of spatial data analysis. The importance of data management to any of the subsequent steps in the analysis should not be underestimated. It is an area where the epidemiologist is confronted with a range of essential concepts, although they may not appear immediately relevant to the intended analytical question.

The specific analytical objectives then lead to three groups of analytical methods: visualization, exploration, and modelling. The first two groups cover techniques that focus solely on examining the spatial dimension of the data. Visualization is probably the most commonly used spatial analysis method, resulting in maps that describe spatial patterns and which are useful for both stimulating more complex analyses and for communicating the results of such analyses. Exploration of spatial data involves the use of statistical methods to determine whether observed patterns are random in space.

Modelling introduces the concept of cause-effect relationships using both spatial and non-spatial data sources to explain or predict spatial patterns. It needs to be emphasized that none of these approaches allows definitive causal inference. There is some overlap among the groups, particularly between visualization and exploration, since meaningful visual presentation may require the use of quantitative analytical methods. The four groups illustrated in Fig. 1.2 can be used to define a logical, sequential process for conducting spatial analyses. It should however be noted that this is not a linear process, as presenting the results from exploration and modelling requires a return to visualization.

1.2 Scientific literature and conferences

The demand for expertise in spatial epidemiological analysis is reflected in the increasing number of textbooks relating to the topic, many of which are aimed at epidemiologists. Bailey and Gatrell (1995) produced one of the first books on spatial data analysis; a comprehensive and practical text that attempted to minimize the use of mathematical theory so that the methods might become more widely accessible. Cressie (1993) is a standard spatial analysis text but with a more mathematical emphasis. More recently, several authors have produced

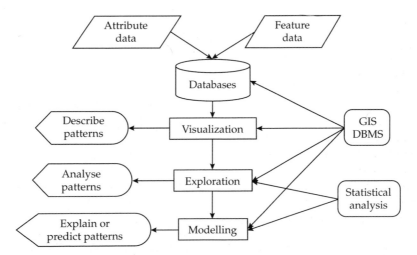

Figure 1.2 Conceptual framework of spatial epidemiological data analysis (GIS = geographic information systems, DBMS = database management system).

books on specific aspects of spatial data analysis, such as Diggle (2003) on the analysis of point patterns, Lawson and Williams (2001) on basic aspects of disease mapping, and both Lawson et al. (2003) and Banerjee et al. (2004) on modelling of spatial data. Others, such as Haining (2003), Waller and Gotway (2004), Schabenberger and Gotway (2005), and Lawson (2006a) have covered the whole subject area. There have also been several textbooks that are collections of chapters authored by different experts in the field (Elliott et al. 1992a; Gatrell and Löytönen 1998; Lawson et al. 1999a; Elliott et al. 2000; Lawson and Denison 2002; Durr and Gatrell 2004; Lawson and Kleinman 2005a; Hay et al. 2006). Despite these developments, general epidemiology texts typically do not include even a basic introduction to spatial analysis, apart from using maps to show disease distribution.

There are an increasing number of peer-reviewed scientific publications that specifically use spatial analysis methods. While these have tended to be primarily visualizations of disease distributions, the use of spatial cluster detection methods has now become a common analytical tool, with the application of spatial modelling techniques lagging somewhat behind. Clearly, this gradient in frequency of application of spatial analysis techniques is also related to the robustness and complexity of the methods, as well as to differences in access to user-friendly tools for performing the analyses. *The International Journal of Health Geographics*[2] is the first peer-reviewed journal that specializes in spatial epidemiology.

The exchange of knowledge resulting from the application of spatial analysis techniques to epidemiological research is also being facilitated by specialist scientific conferences. In the veterinary field, the GisVet[3] conference series provides a forum for the presentation and discussion of scientific developments related to spatial epidemiology. The first conference was held in 2001 in Lancaster, UK, the second in 2004 in Guelph, Canada, and the most recent in 2007 in Copenhagen, Denmark. A new initiative has been the OIE International Conference: Use of GIS in Veterinary Activities[4]

which was held for the first time in 2006 in Silvi Marina, Italy. In the medical field, probably due to the larger volume of research activity, there are no specific spatial analysis conferences, but in most years several one-off scientific meetings are held, such as the Spatial Epidemiology Conference[5] in London in 2006 or The Urban and Regional Information Systems Association's (URISA) GIS in Public Health Conference[6] in 2007.

1.3 Software

The availability of increasingly user-friendly GIS and spatial analysis software has made spatial analysis more accessible to epidemiologists and other researchers. Most advances have occurred in relation to the functionality and variety of GIS software, whereas spatial statistical analysis still necessitates the use of a range of software tools, many of which require some level of programming expertise. Freely available online mapping tools such as Google Earth[7] and Microsoft Virtual Earth[8] have made descriptive interactive mapping accessible to everyone with access to the Internet. The Food and Agriculture Organization of the United Nations (FAO) provides an interactive online mapping system, the Global Livestock Production and Health Atlas (GLiPHA)[9], which focuses on a wide range of livestock-related production and health data for all countries of the world (Clements et al. 2002).

It is useful to distinguish between mapping and GIS software. The former only produces maps and usually has limited data input functionality, whereas the latter provides a whole range of functions that can be broadly categorized into data input, management, analysis, and presentation (Pfeiffer and Hugh-Jones 2002). Examples of mapping software packages include Microsoft MapPoint[10], the free software ArcExplorer[11], and EpiMap[12], which is part of the public domain software package

---

[2] http://www.ij-healthgeographics.com
[3] http://www.gisvet.org
[4] http://www.gisconference.it

[5] http://www.spatepiconf.org
[6] http://www.urisa.org/conferences/health
[7] http://earth.google.com
[8] http://www.microsoft.com/virtualearth/default.aspx
[9] http://www.fao.org/ag/aga/glipha/index.jsp
[10] http://www.microsoft.com/mappoint
[11] http://www.esri.com/software/arcexplorer
[12] http://www.cdc.gov/epiinfo

EpiInfo. GIS software includes ArcGIS by ESRI[13] (probably the most commonly used commercial software package), the IDRISI software from Clark Labs[14] and the open source application GRASS[15], as well as numerous others (see for example, those listed on Wikipedia[16]).

Most of the modern GIS software can handle both vector and raster data sources (defined in Chapter 2), and are also capable of accessing non-spatial relational databases. The ability of GIS to perform spatial analyses varies substantially, and the IDRISI software is probably most comprehensive in this respect. Software such as ERDAS Imagine and ER Mapper, both now owned by Leica Geosystems[17], focus on processing remotely sensed imagery.

Specialized spatial analysis software includes the commercial product ClusterSeer[18] and the public domain software SaTScan[19], which allow for spatial and space–time cluster analyses. GeoDa[20] is also in the public domain and offers a wide range of exploratory data analysis methods for area data, as well as basic mapping capabilities. A wide range of resources for analysing spatial data based on the R programming language and environment for statistical computing and graphics[21] are described on the R Spatial Projects website[22]. Many new developments in statistical spatial analysis first become available as R code. S+SpatialStats is a module of the commercial S-Plus software[23] that allows for exploration and modelling of spatial data. It is based on the public domain code for spatial point-pattern analysis in S-Plus (SPLANCS) which has also been adapted for use in R[24]. The free OpenBUGS[25] software provides specialist tools for performing complex Bayesian modelling of spatial data.

1.4 Spatial data

The increased availability of georeferenced data has facilitated the ascent of spatial epidemiological analysis. An essential requirement of such analyses is georeferenced numerator and denominator data at a spatial resolution sufficiently high to allow meaningful inferences to be made. While it has always been possible to collect such data as part of specific studies (including those based on routine disease surveillance), often such data have either not existed or not been made widely available. Advances in hardware and software development now allow for routine processing of high-resolution data for the purposes of management and simple descriptive analyses by local administrative authorities. Access to such data for research purposes varies among countries due to different data protection and confidentiality legislation, with the latter tending to be more restrictive for human than for animal health problems (Elliott and Wartenberg 2004).

While the available data have increased, so too has the number of data sources, with data quality varying between both datasets and data sources. Efforts are being made to standardize formats and quality[26] and to facilitate access through online geographical data portals, such as FAO's GeoNetwork[27] or the United States government's geodata.gov website[28]. While it is usually possible to obtain various statistics at a national level for most countries, higher-resolution, sub-national data are harder to come by. Unfortunately, it is usually high-resolution data that are needed in order to perform *meaningful* spatial analyses. In such situations it may be necessary to use predicted densities such as FAO's series of livestock density maps with global coverage, the *Gridded Livestock of the World*[29] (Robinson et al. 2007; Wint and Robinson 2007) or its human equivalent, the *Gridded Population of the World* with urban reallocation[30].

Many data sources are generated either by government organizations or those closely linked to

---

[13] http://www.esri.com
[14] http://www.clarklabs.org
[15] http://en.wikipedia.org/wiki/GRASS_GIS
[16] http://en.wikipedia.org/wiki/List_of_GIS_software
[17] http://gi.leica-geosystems.com
[18] http://www.terraseer.com
[19] http://www.satscan.org
[20] https://www.geoda.uiuc.edu
[21] http://www.r-project.org
[22] http://www.sal.uiuc.edu/csiss/Rgeo
[23] http://www.insightful.com
[24] http://www.maths.lancs.ac.uk/Software/Splancs
[25] http://mathstat.helsinki.fi/openbugs

[26] http://www.opengeospatial.org
[27] http://www.fao.org/geonetwork
[28] http://www.geodata.gov
[29] http://www.fao.org/ag/AGAinfo/resources/en/glw/default.html
[30] http://sedac.ciesin.columbia.edu/gpw

government, such as cadastral, postal, meteorological, or national census statistics organizations. Most of these organizations charge for data provision, but also aim to improve and maintain a high standard of data quality. An important component of data cost is associated with updating, particularly if it relates, for example, to cadastral information. Remotely sensed data sources used for describing environmental variables can be updated almost in real time at a relatively modest cost. The wide availability of low-cost global positioning systems (GPS) now allows field-collected data to be readily georeferenced.

1.5 Book content and structure

Consistent with the conceptual framework for spatial epidemiological analysis presented in Fig. 1.2 the book chapters can be grouped into four sections: the first addressing spatial data (Chapter 2), the second introducing visualization (Chapter 3), the third covering exploratory analysis (Chapters 4, 5, and 6), and the fourth presenting analytical techniques used for modelling relationships among diseases and risk factors in the context of risk assessment and decision support (Chapters 7 and 8). The book provides an overview of the range of methods available in spatial epidemiology, with a relatively detailed introduction to the most important methods. The link between spatial epidemiological investigations and policy development is given particular emphasis.

Although readers are expected to have an understanding of quantitative epidemiological concepts, most of the techniques introduced in this book can be applied without having to write complex programming code in specialized software. While it is recognized that the application of statistical techniques requires knowledge of their assumptions, limitations, and interpretation of the outputs, it is hoped that the material presented in the book will encourage interested epidemiologists to explore the different methods further. Waller and Gotway (2004) recognize the need to achieve an appropriate balance between theory and practical application with such a textbook, and warn of the risks associated with such an approach in that the methods

may be inappropriately used and thereby lead to incorrect inferences. Although *Spatial Analysis in Epidemiology* focuses on application rather than theory, it is hoped that by providing a practical, comprehensive, and up-to-date overview of the use of spatial statistics in epidemiology, an appropriate balance has been achieved.

1.5.1 Datasets used

1.5.1.1 *Bovine tuberculosis data*
As part of its intention to focus on application rather than theory, the book includes many worked examples in order to demonstrate the use of the various techniques described. The majority of these examples are based on data collected from Great Britain's cattle population as part of the national bovine tuberculosis (TB) control programme, comprising cattle TB data from 1986 to 1999. This dataset was chosen because it is georeferenced, includes all cattle herds within the country, contains substantial spatial variation in herd density and disease risk, includes a temporal dimension, and disease risk is known to be associated with environmental variables and factors such as presence of local wildlife reservoir species and cattle movement. The data records specify whether a herd was found to have animals reacting positively to the TB test during a particular year. The interval between herd tests varies across the country, ranging from several tests per year to once every four years, depending on disease risk within the region and the disease history of individual herds.

1.5.1.2 *Environmental data*
Chapter 7 reviews analytical methods for exploring factors associated with disease. Table 1.1, adapted from Robinson et al. (2007), provides an overview of some of the types of spatial environmental variables that may be important in such analyses.

Wint et al. (2002) use a comprehensive list of variables in an analysis of environmental correlates for bovine TB. The examples presented in this book use a reduced set of those variables in order to simplify the modelling and to aid comparison of results. In addition to positional information and elevation (obtained from the global GTOPO30 1 km resolution elevation surface, produced by the Global Land

Table 1.1 Generic list of environmental variables relevant to epidemiological analysis

Generic type	Variables
Location	Longitude, latitude
Anthropogenic	Distance to roads
	Distance to city lights
Demographic	Human population
Topographic	Elevation
Land cover	Normalized Difference Vegetation Index (NDVI)[a-c]
Temperature	Land surface temperature[a-e]
	Air temperature[f]
	Middle infrared reflectance[a]
Water and moisture	Vapour pressure deficit (VPD)[a-c]
	Distance to rivers
	Cold cloud duration[a]
	Potential evapotranspiration[g]
General climatic	Modelled length of growing period[g]

[a] Hay (2000); [b] Green and Hay (2002); [c] Hay et al. (2006); [d] Hay and Lennon (1999); [e] Price (1984); [f] Goetz et al. (2000); [g] Fischer at al. (2002)

Information System of the United States Geological Survey, Earth Resources Observation Systems Data Centre), a series of 1 km satellite-derived variables was obtained from the Advanced Very High Resolution Radiometer (AVHRR) on board the National Oceanographic and Atmospheric Administration (NOAA) series of satellites. Decadal (ten-day) composite images were obtained from 1992/1993 and 1995/1996, and combined into monthly averages to provide complete temporal coverage of a nominal calendar year. The channel data were converted into five estimates of geophysical variables (Table 1.1): (1) Normalized Difference Vegetation Index (NDVI)—an estimate of vegetation activity, whose integrated value relates to primary production over a specified period (Tucker and Sellers 1986); (2) land surface temperature, (3) air temperature, (4) middle infrared reflectance taken from Channel 3 of the NOAA-AVHRR—a temperature-related variable that is useful in discriminating between different land-covers, and (5) vapour pressure deficit (VPD)—an estimate of atmospheric humidity near the earth's surface indicative of the 'drying power' of air.

Each time series was subjected to temporal Fourier processing (named after the French mathematician, Joseph Fourier), and re-sampled and re-projected to match the bovine TB dataset. The Fourier processing of satellite data, described in detail in Rogers et al. (1996) is of great value to epidemiological investigations since it reveals the seasonal characteristics of the environment. Each multi-temporal series is reduced to seven separate data layers: the mean, the phases and amplitudes of the annual, bi-annual, and tri-annual cycles of change. These are supplemented by three additional variables: the minimum, maximum, and variance of the satellite-derived geophysical variables. Collectively, these numerical indictors of the level (mean, minimum, maximum), timing (phase), seasonality (amplitude), and variability (variance) of each satellite-derived environmental variable give a unique 'fingerprint' of habitat type; they provide a link between the satellite signal and biological processes that determine the epidemiology of the disease. A further advantage of the Fourier processing is that it reduces the vast number of individual decadal images to a manageable and relatively independent set of variables, more amenable to statistical analysis and interpretation.

The power of these Fourier-processed data to distinguish habitat types is illustrated in Fig. 1.3,

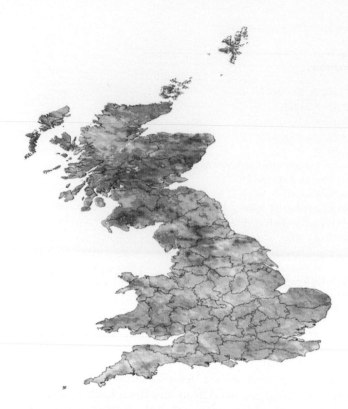

Figure 1.3 False colour composite of Fourier-processed air temperature variables for Great Britain. The average value (the 'zero-order' component) is displayed in red, the phase of the first-order component is displayed in green, and the amplitude of the first-order component is displayed in blue (this caption refers to the colour version of the figure which can be found in the plate section). See plate 1.

a false colour composite of Fourier-processed air temperature variables for Great Britain. The average value (the 'zero-order' component) is displayed in red, the phase of the first-order component is displayed in green, and the amplitude of the first-order component is displayed in blue. Broad regional differences can be seen, such as the predominance of red in the south, indicating relatively high and less variable average temperatures, and the predominance of blue and green to the north indicating greater variability in average temperatures and later seasons, respectively.

In addition to the generic variable types listed in Table 1.1., analysis of different diseases may require other more specifically relevant variables. In the case of the bovine TB examples used throughout the book variables such as herd size, cattle density, proportion of dairy cattle, and abundance of potential wild hosts of disease, such as badgers, may also be important correlates of disease presence.

CHAPTER 2

Spatial data

2.1 Introduction

Data collected for the purpose of epidemiological investigations typically focus on the attributes of observations such as the disease status of individual animals. If coordinate locations are also recorded, the spatial pattern of the epidemiological problem can be investigated, in addition to classical risk factor analyses. The presence of a geographical reference for each observation firstly allows for analyses incorporating geographical relationships between the observations and their attributes, and secondly, additional attribute data can be obtained by linking spatially to other georeferenced data. Investigations aimed at describing and understanding the processes that influence the occurrence of disease can benefit greatly from access to digital information systems that can represent the environment within which these processes operate. A key component of such systems is representation of the space dimension. They often also reflect time but this is usually done as an attribute of spatial entities. Due to the complexity of the real world any such digital representation is an abstraction, often involving substantial generalization and simplification (Haining 2003).

2.2 Spatial data and GIS

Data georeferenced with point locations, for example, households or cattle farms, can be managed by any database management system by adding two data columns; one for the x- and one for the y-coordinate. A simple 'map' can be produced using scatterplot graph functions in electronic spreadsheets. If the boundaries of administrative areas are also to be shown, more specialized applications are required, such as mapping software or GIS, which are capable of accurately representing the relative geographical position of different types of (otherwise often unrelated) information. It is then possible to produce a map showing the point locations together with, for example, contour lines expressing elevation above sea-level, as well as other data such as rivers, roads, and railway lines.

GIS are now used in many different areas including town planning, ecology, and utility management, reflecting the importance of the spatial dimension to most processes occurring in the world around us. GIS technology has a hardware, software, and organizational component (Burrough and McDonnell 1998), which must be balanced appropriately. This means that the computer hardware, including any input and output devices, needs to be able to cope with the data volumes and computational requirements. The software application should have functions for the collection, storage, manipulation, analysis, and presentation of spatial data. However, neither of the two components (hardware and software) is sufficient if the system is not placed in a suitable organizational context with appropriately skilled operators. Many GIS are now available and, through increased demand and widespread use, have become increasingly user-friendly, with greater functionality and a greater capacity to store and manipulate different spatial data types. At its core, GIS software has a database capable of handling georeferenced information, complemented by a series of software tools responsible for the input, management, and analysis of data, and the production of maps and related output.

2.2.1 Data types

Several conceptual models can be used to represent a geographical space. The two extremes are *entities* and *fields*. The first approach views space as being occupied by entities with specific attributes, and their position can be mapped using geographical coordinates. The second describes the variation in a particular attribute value in space as a continuous mathematical function or field. The choice of the appropriate approach depends on the data and their intended use. The continuous field would be more suitable for investigating spatial processes whereas entities should be used for administrative purposes (Burrough and McDonnell 1998). Typical representations of entities in GIS are points, lines, and polygons. Points may define, for example, the geographic locations of infected animals. Lines can represent linear features such as roads and rivers. Polygons are used to define contiguous areas that have a common characteristic, for example, they may represent administrative areas, land parcels owned by the same person, or areas of a certain vegetation or soil type. All entity data types have associated attributes. For example, the attribute data for the point location mentioned above is that it relates to an infected animal, and may include other attributes such as the animal species and

type of disease. Continuous fields, which include the spatial patterns of rainfall, temperature, or elevation, normally have only a single attribute.

The representation of these conceptual data models within a GIS can be in vector, raster, or triangulated irregular network (TIN) format (Zeiler 1999) (Fig. 2.1). Vectors represent shapes of spatial features based on an ordered set of coordinates linked to potentially multiple attribute values. They are particularly suitable for describing entities such as points, lines, or polygons. With spatial data stored in vector format it is possible to perform geometric calculations, such as length and area, as well as to describe proximity. Vectors are used to define, for example, the locations of infected herds, as well as of administrative boundaries. Raster format uses a two-dimensional grid to represent spatial data, and is well suited to describing continuous fields. Each cell has a single attribute which is the value of the spatial phenomenon being described, such as elevation above sea level, total monthly rainfall, or average monthly temperature. The value represents a summary function of the variation

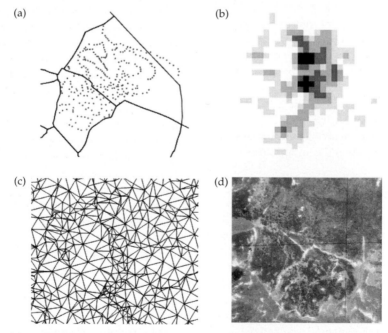

(a)　　　　　　　　　　(b)

(c)　　　　　　　　　　(d)

Figure 2.1 Examples of data representation in GIS (all based on data from a field study of TB in wild possums in New Zealand). (a) A vector map defining paddock boundaries and locations of traps, (b) a raster map showing density of possum captures, (c) a triangulated irregular network (TIN) structure based on the digital elevation model for the study site, and (d) an aerial photograph of the study site.

in the attribute within the area described by the cell. Although smaller cell sizes allow for a better description of the spatial variation in attribute values, they increase the digital storage space and processing power required. The TIN structure is used to represent three-dimensional surfaces. It is based on a set of integrated nodes with elevation values and triangles. This format allows analyses to be performed that require, for example, identification of watersheds. It is also used to interpolate elevation values for any location within the extent defined by the TIN. While raster format can also be used for this purpose, the advantage of a TIN is that it allows for varying data density depending on the detail required to accurately represent a surface.

Attribute information for spatial entities can be generated based on relationships defined in the GIS data model. These include topological, spatial, and general relationships. Topological relationships allow quick identification of neighbouring land parcels. Spatial relationships involve operations among different layers of spatial data and allow for the calculation of, for example, the area occupied by different vegetation or soil types on a farm, or the distance to the nearest road or river. General relationships need to be explicitly defined as they cannot be inferred from the geographical position of the relevant entities. This includes linkages to internal and external database tables.

2.2.2 Data storage and interchange

Storage of attribute data can be in a simple tabular or a more complex format, based on relational or object-oriented data models. In most GIS, entity data has a unique key variable (Fig. 2.2a) that allows linkage to other data tables containing further attribute information for each entity. These can be part of the GIS or may be external to it, and are accessed using data query languages such as the Structured Query Language (SQL). Examples of attribute data linked to a farm and georeferenced through the point location of the main farmhouse include information such as the national herd identification number, name of the owner, address, and postcode (Fig. 2.2b). While these data may already be stored in the GIS together with the spatial data, further attribute data can be added through a relational link from external databases via the herd identification number (Fig. 2.2c). This would give access to, for example, TB-test results from the national TB-testing database, the number of cows purchased and sold during the previous twelve months from national animal movement databases, and the mortality of calves during the same time period from animal identification databases.

Spatial data are most commonly organized as layers or coverages, each describing a particular theme such as rainfall or farm boundaries. Recently, object-oriented geographic data models have been developed, of which ESRI's geodatabase is an example. One of the advantages of this new approach is that, in contrast to coverages, it does not require separation of the real world into distinct themes, each stored, manipulated, and updated separately, and requiring relatively complex tools to link them back together for purposes of analysis.

The interchange of spatial data between software-specific formats is often complex. The availability of formats, such as ESRI's shape file format,

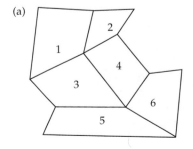

Figure 2.2 Linking entities on a farm map with multiple data tables via herd ID. (a) Farm boundary map, (b) farm data table, and (c) animal data table.

has made this easier as any software product can include procedures that read and write to that format. Data conversion among vector, raster, and TIN formats is sometimes associated with a loss in data quality due to the compromises that have to be made when, for example, converting a river network into a raster map, as a straight vector line can fairly accurately represent a river but if it is converted into a set of raster cells, resolution will be lost unless very small raster cells are used. In addition, attribute data, such as direction and rate of flow of the river, would be less readily represented in raster format (see Fig. 2.3). A TIN can be generated from vector data representing point elevation values. Its disadvantage is that specialized procedures are required to generate the TIN, and to make full use of its particular strengths. Some formats are better suited to particular types of data and it is best to maintain the appropriate format as far as possible. Often though, analyses require data to be in the same format, meaning that data quality must be compromised.

2.2.3 Data collection and management

The collection of spatial data involves capture, verification, and a structuring process (Burrough and McDonnell 1998). Digital data can be obtained from a supplier, digitized from paper maps or scanned images, derived from manually collected field data, or interpolated from digital point values. During field surveys, the use of electronic means of data recording, such as GPS technology, allows very precise locational information to be obtained. Optical and digital remote sensing by aircraft or satellites can provide data ranging from photographic representations of particular geographical areas, ground reflectivity or emissivity for defined ranges of wavelengths of the electromagnetic spectrum, to information on surface elevation and surface material density and texture. The spatial resolution of commercial satellite imagery is now as high as 15 m (for LandSat 7) on the ground. Data capture should be followed by verification which can be achieved, for example, through comparison with paper maps or by 'ground truthing'. Data structuring is the final activity during data collection and refers to the procedures involved in appropriately formatting the captured data. Examples include geometric or radiometric correction of remotely sensed data, conversion of reflectance or emittance values to geophysical values such as temperature or vegetation indices, or conversion from one data format to another, such as from raster to vector, in order to produce a database suitable for its intended use.

In order to integrate data effectively, a common spatial reference frame must be defined for all spatial data to be used in a particular project. This is provided by a coordinate system, but it is also possible to convert between different systems. Most systems are based on plane, orthogonal Cartesian coordinates. Almost every country has its own regional system with its own origin so that local distortions are minimized and the use of coordinates with unnecessarily large numbers is avoided. The spatial units are usually metric units of distance or decimal degrees. The latitude-longitude system allows geographic position to be expressed anywhere around the world. The longitude (east–west) and latitude (north–south) positions express location relative

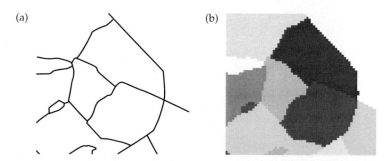

(a)   (b)

Figure 2.3 Conversion from vector to raster map. (a) The initial vector map, and (b) the raster map derived from the vector map.

to the Greenwich Meridian and Equator, respectively. The process of representing locations on the globe on a plane surface requires the use of mathematical expressions of the Earth's curvature called ellipsoids. Ellipsoids may also take account of the flattening that occurs at the poles. Cylindrical, conical, or azimuthal projections are then used to project geographic locations from a specific ellipsoid on to a plane surface. This process always results in some distortion which becomes particularly apparent when large areas or countries, such as China or the Russian Federation, are presented. Different projections have been designed for different purposes. Some preserve area, some preserve distance, and others preserve shape (angle). Choice of an appropriate projection therefore depends on the application. For example, equal-area projections are often considered important in remotely sensed data so that each pixel represents the same area on the ground. The simplest projection is the geographic or Plate Carrée projection, in which points of longitude and latitude are plotted directly on a regular grid. The lines of longitude (meridians) on the graph are spaced the same distance apart as the lines of latitude (parallels), thus forming squares. This simple representation does not preserve area, distance, or shape but is the most widely used projection in the collection, storage, and interchange of data. Another commonly used projection, on which most national topographic maps are based, is the Universal Transverse Mercator (UTM) coordinate system, developed by the United States military. It divides the world into 60 grid zones, each divided into a northern and southern part, and the coordinates of any point can be expressed in terms of metres from the origin (bottom left hand corner) of the grid zone in which it falls (Banerjee et al. 2004). Useful references to the theory and application of map projections include Snyder (1987) and Canters and DeClair (1989).

Geographic scale typically refers to the resolution at which spatial data are captured and presented, and inferences drawn from any analyses need to consider the original scale of the data. It is one of the dangers of GIS that the original spatial data can be manipulated so that they appear to have a higher resolution than that at which the original measurements were made.

Data are often obtained from a multitude of sources and, in order for them to be used appropriately by investigators other than the original data collectors, they should be accompanied by descriptive metadata that summarize their lineage and content. Metadata include information on the data source, date collected, any data manipulations performed as well as, for example, the coordinate system, resolution, and data model (Longley et al. 2001). The creation of metadata can be a time-consuming and expensive process and is often neglected, but it is becoming increasingly important due to the widespread dissemination of datasets over the internet and the explosive increase in the quantity of georeferenced data sources.

2.2.4 Data quality

Both the choice of representation and the accuracy of the measurements affect how well spatial data reflect the real world (Haining 2003). The choice of representation includes the type of data format selected, for example vector versus raster, or point versus area, as well as the methods of attribute measurement such as through remote sensing or continuous recording at meteorological stations. Assessment of data quality needs to consider the accuracy of both the location information and of the attribute values.

Ideally location of farms should be represented as polygons reflecting the property boundaries of individual farms. Usually, this is considered to be too costly and would require more complex analytical procedures, particularly if a farm includes several non-contiguous land parcels. In such instances farms are more easily represented as single point locations. The decision then has to be made whether to use the geographical coordinates of the farmhouse, or those of the centroid calculated from the main farm area. Disadvantages of condensing a farm's area into a single point-location include the fact that any neighbourhood calculations have to be based on distance rather than true property boundary adjacency and, in terms of analysis, the assumption is then made that all farm properties are circular. It is also likely to bias the results of any statistical analyses since these methods typically assume that centroids represent precise locations of the events of interest (Jacquez and Jacquez 1999). Durr and Froggatt (2002) analyse the impact of using different methods for representing farm properties and conclude that single point-locations are the most cost-effective method.

Epidemiological interpretation of disease surveillance data requires access to, and information on, the spatial distribution of an appropriate denominator. Ideally the locations of all livestock holdings around the country would be available, or at least summary estimates at some administrative level of aggregation, for example, county or parish in Great Britain. Most surveillance data are currently presented as tabulated, summary statistics generated at a defined administrative level of aggregation such as district or province. These data can easily be presented using a GIS, since the boundaries of these administrative units are available in digital formats for most countries in the world. However, it is important to match the level of administrative aggregation with the spatial resolution at which epidemiological inferences are to be drawn. For example, in order to make a broad assessment of the occurrence of bovine TB in Great Britain, aggregation at the county level could be acceptable. Alternatively, if clusters resulting from point sources of infection were to be identified, it would be necessary to work with data aggregated at a much higher resolution or ideally with individual farm locations. It is also important to recognize that changing levels of data aggregation may result in very different observed spatial patterns. This process has been called the modifiable areal unit problem (MAUP), and it is similar to the 'ecological fallacy' in epidemiology; a widely recognized error in the interpretation of statistical data whereby inferences about the nature of individuals are based upon aggregate statistics collected for the group to which those individuals belong (Cressie 1993).

When using GIS data, it is important to recognize that they always contain errors, resulting from factual mistakes or from measurement variability. If these errors are not considered during spatial analyses, regardless of whether the latter involve Boolean or numerical operations, the consequences are unpredictable due to the propagation of errors. The impact of uncertainty in the context of quantitative spatial analysis can be assessed using Monte Carlo simulation (see Chapter 4) or analytical approaches (Burrough and McDonnell 1998).

2.3 Spatial effects

2.3.1 Spatial heterogeneity and dependence

The basic principle of spatial dependence is that attribute values measured at locations close together are more similar than those from more distant locations. If this dependence does not vary (i.e. is the same for any location in a geographic area), the spatial process is termed stationary. If on the other hand, the dependence structure varies throughout the area, the process is termed non-stationary or heterogeneous. If the dependence in a stationary process is only affected by distance, but not direction, then it is considered to be isotropic, whereas if the dependence is different in different directions, it is considered to be anisotropic.

The total variation amongst attribute values of a spatial process is the result of large (macro-) and medium/small (meso-/micro-) scale variation (Cressie 1993; Haining 2003). They are usually measured on a continuous scale, and have also been called first- and second-order spatial effects (Bailey and Gatrell 1995). Macro-scale variation expresses itself as a trend across a geographical region. For example, risk of disease may increase from south to north in a region as a result of differences in temperature affecting survival of an infectious organism. Meso-scale variation on the other hand describes the local dependence of a spatial process, also called spatial heterogeneity. This could express itself, for example, as clusters of an infectious disease around livestock markets, or local habitat preferences for a disease vector. One of the two types typically dominates the observed spatial variation; which it is depends heavily on the scale and extent at which observations are made. Most of the currently available statistical analysis methods only allow one of these effects to be modelled, and may produce biased results if both are present and standard fixed-effect modelling methods are used.

2.3.2 Edge effects

The boundaries or edges of an area may be the result of physical barriers such as the sea, or may be defined boundaries such as the borders of administrative regions (e.g. country or county) or study areas. Data for the area beyond the edges are frequently either incomplete, unavailable (e.g. a different country), or non-existent (e.g. when the sea is the boundary). Points (or area units) near these edges, are therefore likely to have fewer neighbours than those in the centre of the study area. This presents a problem when performing calculations that borrow strength from neighbouring areas (such as kernel smoothing, see Chapter 6) or when investigating data for the presence of clustering (Chapters 4 and 5), as the fewer neighbours may distort any estimates for points (or area units) near the edges. These distortions are referred to as edge effects. Although edge effects may be negligible when dealing with large-scale effects, they can be considerable when estimating small-scale effects close to the boundary. Edge effects are usually dealt with either by using a weighting system that gives less weight to those observations near the boundary, or through the use of guard areas (Lawson et al. 1999b)

2.3.3 Representing neighbourhood relationships

Continuity and connectivity are typical characteristics of spatial processes known as topology. With raster data, topology is implicitly defined in the data through the relative positioning of individual cells within the regular grid. The situation is more complex for vector data and different methods can be used to describe topology. In the simplest case only the spatial coordinates are stored, and the neighbourhood relationships are derived during a database query or as part of a statistical analysis procedure. In the case of polygon data it is possible to store topological information (i.e. which boundaries are shared by which polygons) directly with the data.

One of the defining characteristics of GIS software is that it can generate new data based on transformations and queries of existing data, taking into account topological and spatial relationships. Distance and area calculations can be performed on raster or vector data. Slope and aspect can be derived from raster or TIN presentations of digital elevation models. Buffer areas around spatial entities can be defined, for example, to identify herds within a specified distance of an infected herd that ought to be tested for the presence of disease. Overlay operations use spatial relationships among different layers of geographic data. These can involve either simple Boolean or more complex mathematical operations. One example is the GIS point-in-polygon operation that can be used, for example, to count the number of diseased herds (defined by point locations) within an administrative area (defined as a polygon). Another example is the polygon overlay function, which could be used to calculate the proportion of total forest area on each farm in a region derived from farm boundary and vegetation type polygon layers. It is also possible to create new polygon layers including, for example, all contiguous land parcels belonging to the same farm, by merging individual polygons from a land parcel map based on landowner identification (Longley et al. 2001).

Statistical methods that take into account spatial dependence require a spatial weights matrix to be generated that describes how the observations in a dataset are related to each other. Different types of matrices can be calculated. A binary contiguity matrix describes whether or not spatial objects, such as farms, are neighbours. These can be extended from first-order to multiple-order adjacencies. The information stored in matrices can also be more complex, for example, parameters such as distance, or length of a common border (Haining 2003).

2.3.4 Statistical significance testing with spatial data

Independence of observations is a fundamental assumption of most classical statistical procedures using hypothesis testing based on theoretical, large sample (asymptotic) sampling distributions. If spatial dependence is present in a dataset, this assumption is violated. In this case, data from geographically close observations contribute less additional information than they would if they were further apart. A potential consequence of ignoring this effect in a statistical analysis is to underestimate errors and to overestimate statistical significance levels, thereby increasing the risk of making a Type I error. Different approaches can be used to deal with this problem in hypothesis testing. The simplest is to reduce the effective sample size (Haining 2003). Some statistical software packages such as SAS[31] for Windows Version 9 (SAS Institute, Cary, North Carolina) and OpenBUGS[32] (Spiegelhalter et al. 2003) allow modelling of the dependence structure as part of the error variance in a statistical model (Haining 2003; Lawson et al. 2003; Banerjee et al. 2004). This method is implemented in generalized linear modelling approaches based on maximum-likelihood or Bayesian estimation. A conceptually simple method for hypothesis testing that is not adversely affected by spatial dependence is Monte Carlo randomization (Dwass 1957). This approach produces null hypothesis distributions based on repeated randomizations of the data used in the analysis. The individual values of the test statistic calculated for each randomization are then used together to represent the null hypothesis distribution, against which the observed value of the test statistic is compared, and a p-value calculated (Fortin and Jacquez 2000). This method requires large numbers of randomizations, and can be computationally demanding if used with large spatial datasets or complex spatial processes (Lawson 2001a).

Song and Kulldorff (2003) show how the statistical power of spatial analysis methods can vary considerably. Some analytical procedures involve multiple tests using the same procedure on the same data, for example when looking for clustering of events, and thus have a high risk of committing a Type I error (Thomas 1985; Haybittle et al. 1995). Bonferroni or Simes p-value adjustments can be used to correct for this effect, resulting in a reduced threshold for significance. It should however be noted that the use of these methods results in a conservative assessment of statistical significance (Perneger 1998).

2.4 Conclusion

The integration of the spatial dimension into epidemiological investigations provides an opportunity for conducting more informative descriptive analyses and gaining additional insights into the causal processes under investigation. However, there is a cost associated with this benefit in the form of additional computer hardware, software, and training. Statistical analysis of spatial data requires the use of specific methods that can take account of the potential presence of dependence as a result of geographical proximity. Although the number of available georeferenced databases has substantially increased and their cost decreased, the often substantial variation in quality between and within spatial databases remains a problem, and therefore access to complete and up-to-date metadata is of particular importance when working with spatial data.

---

[31] http://www.sas.com
[32] http://www.mrc-bsu.cam.ac.uk/bugs

CHAPTER 3

Spatial visualization

3.1 Introduction

One of the first steps in any epidemiological analysis is to visualize the spatial characteristics of a dataset. This allows for an appreciation of any patterns that might be present, identification of obvious errors, and the generation of hypotheses about factors that might influence the observed pattern. Visualization is also important for communicating the findings to the target audience using, for example, maps of a disease distribution, with or without correction for the influence of known confounders. This chapter outlines techniques for visualizing spatial data, and describes methods that might be applied in the early phase of an analysis where the objective is to detect obvious spatial patterns and to screen a dataset for errors. It also considers elements of good cartography and other factors that need to be taken into account when communicating spatial information to a wider audience.

3.2 Point data

Perhaps the oldest and most frequently used method for visualizing point data is to plot the locations of study subjects using their Cartesian coordinates. John Snow's account of the Golden Square cholera epidemic in 1854 bears testimony to the usefulness of this technique, when high numbers of cases of cholera around a public water pump provided powerful support to the hypothesis that the disease was transmitted via contaminated drinking water (Snow 1855; McLeod 2000; Vinten-Johansen et al. 2003; Fig. 1.1). Although point maps are the simplest way to visualize disease event information when the locations of events are known, they present problems where there are either large numbers of events or multiple events at the same location. In such situations the resulting maps tend to be cluttered, making it difficult to appreciate the density of events. Further difficulties with point maps arise when attribute information needs to be displayed at each location. The use of different symbols to represent attribute values is one solution, but large numbers of points and a wide range of attribute values results in a display that is difficult to interpret.

Where there are few locations to be plotted and interest lies simply in showing the location of events rather than the spatial distribution of attribute values, point maps provide a means of presenting the data in its 'raw' format, unmodified by any statistical analysis that might be applied to aid or enhance interpretation. This can be useful for communication. A display of the raw data allows users of the information to appreciate the spatial pattern without being burdened by the technical details of analyses done to facilitate data display. Fig. 3.1 is a map of Great Britain showing the point location of holdings for which TB-positive cattle were identified at slaughter from 1985 to 1997, illustrating that the disease occurred mainly in the southwest of the country.

Kernel smoothing methods are an effective means of visualizing spatial pattern when there are large numbers of events (Chapter 6), as they allow for visualization of both the spatial distribution and the density of events.

3.3 Aggregated data

The process of aggregation involves summarizing a group of individual data points into a single value to produce, for example, a total, mean, median, or standard deviation. This summary statistic may then be assigned a spatial location; often a discrete

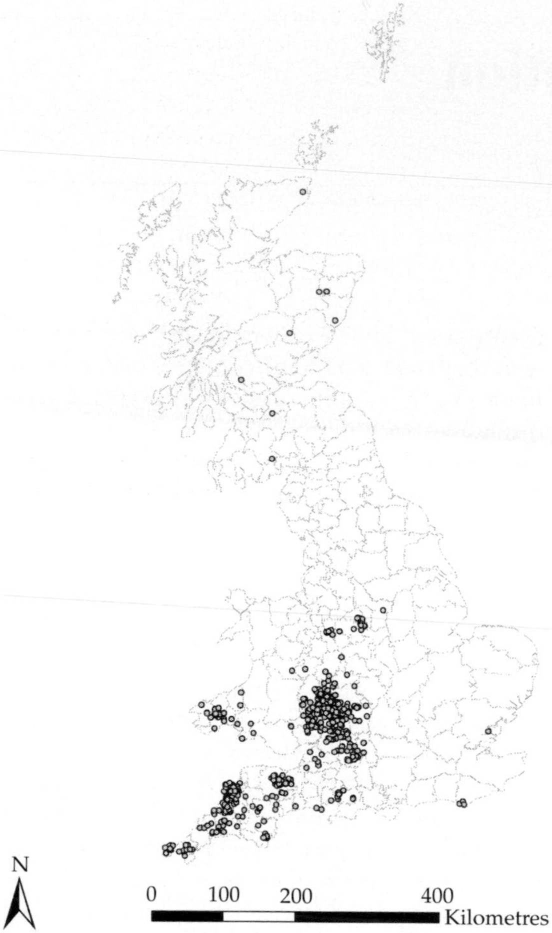

N

Figure 3.1 Point map showing the distribution of holdings in Great Britain for which TB-positive cattle were identified at slaughter in 1985–1997.

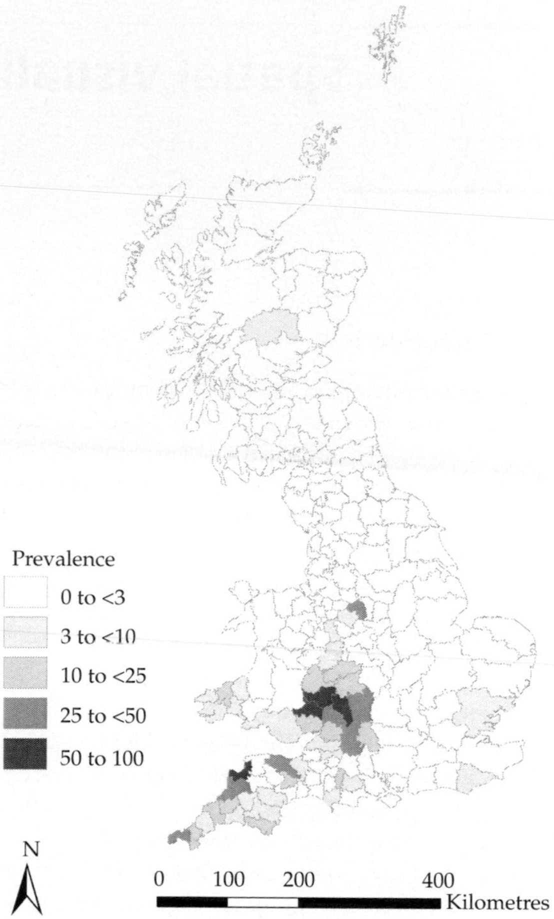

N

Figure 3.2 Choropleth map showing the prevalence of TB-test positive cattle herds in Great Britain (expressed as the number of TB-positive holdings per 100,000 holdings) for 1985–1997.

area such as a state, county, or some other administrative region. In spatial epidemiology, the most common form of data aggregation occurs when counts of disease events within a defined area are summed to yield the total number of disease cases in each area. Disease counts can then be expressed as a function of the population size to provide estimates of prevalence, incidence risk, or incidence rate per unit area. Choropleth maps are the most commonly used means for visualizing data in this format. The term 'choropleth' is derived from the Greek *khoros*, meaning 'place' and *plethein*, meaning 'to be full, or to become full'. Thus, as implied by its Greek

derivative, a choropleth map shows information by 'filling' (colouring) each component area with colour, providing an indication of the magnitude of the variable of interest. Fig. 3.2 is an example of a choropleth map showing the prevalence of TB-test positive cattle herds in Great Britain aggregated by county for 1985 to 1997. This map shows a spatial trend with counties in southwest England and south Wales having a higher prevalence of TB-positive herds than the eastern and northern counties.

Although choropleth maps tend to be the most widely-used method for illustrating the spatial distribution of disease data, they have three inherent problems. Firstly, component polygons of the study region that are large tend to dominate the display and may induce bias in interpretation (Monmonier and De Blij 1996). Secondly, patterns that are observed across zones may be as much a function of the chosen zone boundaries as of the underlying spatial distribution of the attribute of interest, an effect known as the modifiable areal unit problem (MAUP) (Openshaw 1984). The third problem relates to the distribution of the data values being plotted, as highly skewed distributions are difficult to display using a finite number of colour shading scales.

One approach to the problem of physical dominance of large areas is to geometrically transform each of the areas of interest, thereby making its area proportional to the corresponding attribute value but maintaining the spatial contiguity of each area. The result is known as a cartogram (Dorling 1995). Cartograms distort area and distance, forsaking spatial detail, in an effort to display the spatial characteristics of attribute data more effectively. The usual objective is to reveal patterns that might not be readily apparent from a conventional map, or more generally, to improve legibility. Fig. 3.3a shows a map of Great Britain divided into 178 areas, each containing approximately 20,000 head of adult cattle (calculated from agricultural census data collected between 1986 and 1996 (Stevenson et al. 2005). Fig. 3.3b is a cartogram of the same data where area boundaries were distorted so that the size of each area was in proportion to the number of cattle present. From Fig. 3.3b it

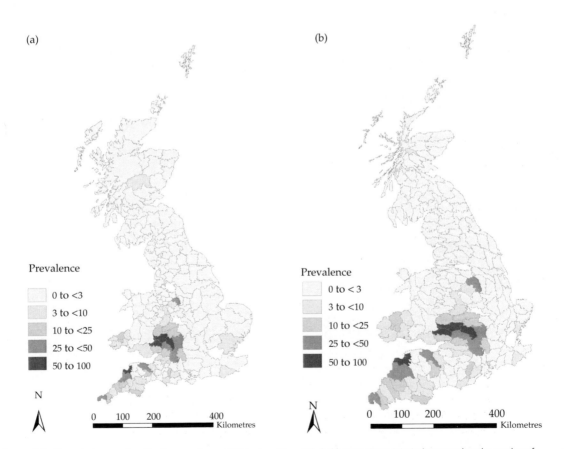

Figure 3.3 Choropleth maps showing the prevalence of TB-test positive cattle holdings in Great Britain (expressed as the number of TB-positive holdings per 100,000 holdings) for 1985–1997. (a) Untransformed area boundaries and (b) a cartogram, where the boundaries of each area have been distorted according to size of cattle population.

is readily apparent that the highest densities of cattle are in the southwest of England and Wales while the east of England and Scotland are areas of relatively low cattle density. The inference we can make from Fig. 3.3b is that the holding-level prevalence of TB is highest in those areas of the country with the greatest numbers of cattle.

Extending the idea of the cartogram further, Selvin et al. (1998) and Schulman et al. (1988) proposed that the size of spatial units within an area of study could be transformed using population counts to yield population density-equalized areas. Plotting the location of disease events over these density-equalized areas allows the spatial distribution of disease events to be visualized, accounting for the (often) irregular spatial distribution of the population at risk. Fig. 3.4 provides an example of this approach. Fig. 3.4a shows the distribution of the 1980 census population of non-Hispanic white females aged between 45 and 64 in Alameda and Contra Costa counties, California. Each dot, plotted at random within its census tract, represents 20 women in this so-called 'dot-density' map. The population is mostly concentrated in a few urban areas. Fig. 3.4b shows the distribution of 68 cases of breast cancer diagnosed between 1968 and 1972, each plotted at random in its census tract of residence. As expected, the distribution of cases in Fig. 3.4b is similar to the distribution of the underlying population at risk (Fig. 3.4a).

In Fig. 3.4c the tract boundaries have been adjusted by a density equalized map projection

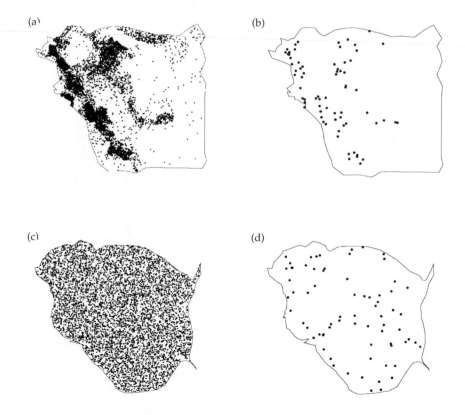

Figure 3.4 Illustration of a density equalized map projection (DEMP) analysis. (a) A dot density map showing the distribution of the 1980 census population of non-Hispanic white females aged between 45 and 64 in Alameda and Contra Costa counties, California. Each dot, plotted at random within its census tract, represents 20 women. (b) The distribution of 68 cases of breast cancer diagnosed between 1968 and 1972, each plotted at random in its census tract of residence. (c) Tract boundaries have been adjusted by a DEMP transformation. (d) The 68 cases of breast cancer plotted at random within the transformed boundaries. Reproduced from Selvin et al. (1998) http://www.merrill.olm.net/mdocs/demp/ with permission from *the American Public Health Association.*

(DEMP) transformation. Again, each dot plotted at random within the transformed boundaries of its census tract represents 20 women. Fig. 3.4c shows that population density has been almost perfectly equalized by the DEMP transformation. In Fig. 3.4d each of the 68 cases is plotted at random within the transformed boundaries of its census tract. Selvin et al. (1998) conclude that there is a hint of non-uniformity in this distribution suggesting that further investigative effort be applied to determine its significance.

With respect to the MAUP, a general rule of practice should be to analyse area data using the smallest area units for which data are available. Aggregation to larger areas should be avoided unless there are good reasons for doing so. Re-analysis of the same dataset using different polygonal boundary definitions is advised, if this is practical (Arlinghaus 1995; Lawson and Williams 2001). Alternatively, irregular area (or point location) data may be re-aggregated to fine, regular lattices, an approach adopted by Abrial et al. (2005) in their analysis of the bovine spongiform encephalopathy (BSE) epidemic in France.

For highly skewed distributions, transformations can be applied to the data. However, in doing so some degree of interpretability is lost since extreme values become truncated (typically) into a single category. Dynamic exploratory spatial data analysis (ESDA) techniques are particularly useful in this situation where conventional graphical data displays, for example histograms or box-and-whisker plots, are presented in conjunction with mapped data on a computer terminal. Using a technique termed 'brushing', data values on the graph are selected interactively and their location displayed simultaneously on the map (Haslett et al. 1991). A variety of software packages with this functionality have been developed including SAGE[33] (Haining et al. 1998) and the GeoDa package[34] (Anselin et al. 2006; Fig. 3.5). The GGobi package[35] (Swayne et al. 1998) allows brushing to

[33] ftp://ftp.shef.ac.uk/pub/uni/academic/D-H/g/sage/sagehtm/sage.htm
[34] https://www.geoda.uiuc.edu
[35] http://www.ggobi.org

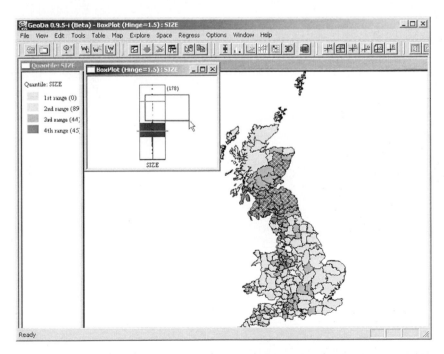

Figure 3.5 Dynamic exploratory spatial data analysis (ESDA) using the GeoDa software. The screen shot shows two windows: (main) a choropleth map of area-level herd size, and (inset) a box-and-whisker plot showing the distributional features of the same data. See plate 2.

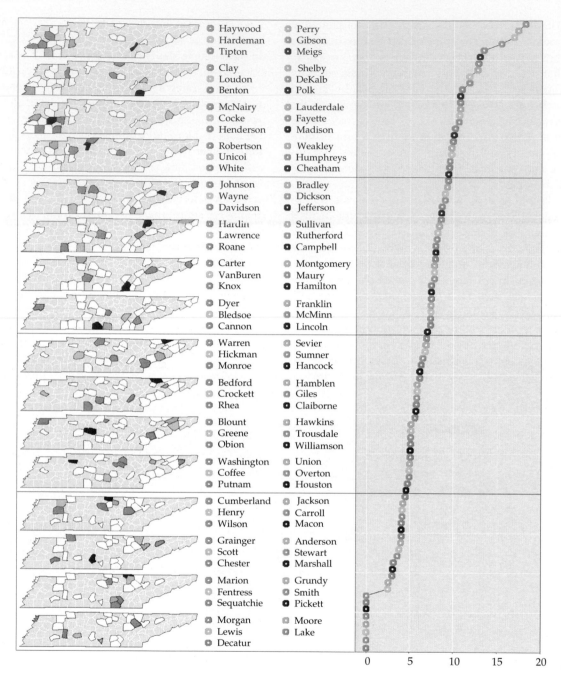

Figure 3.6 Conditioned choropleth map of median infant mortality rate per 1000 births in the state of Tennessee, USA between 1992 and 1997. Reproduced from Carr et al. (2000) with permission from *Statistics in Medicine*. See plate 3.

be carried out on non-spatial data and has been adapted for spatial applications (Symanzik et al. 1998). The technique of 'brushing' is demonstrated using GeoDa in Fig. 3.5 where data points on the box-and-whisker plot, selected interactively by the user, are highlighted simultaneously on the displayed choropleth map. Developing the ESDA technique further, Carr et al. (2000) describe the use of conditioned choropleth maps for demonstrating relationships between a dependent variable, represented in a classed choropleth map, and explanatory variables represented as a scatterplot or error-bar plot. The conditioned choropleth map in Fig. 3.6 shows an aggregation of counties with relatively high median infant mortality rates in the far west of the state of Tennessee, USA. A key feature of conditioned choropleth maps is that they allow the distributional form of the mapped variable to be shown in a static display (unlike the dynamic exploratory approach shown in Fig. 3.5, which is really only effective for communication when it is used interactively with a computer).

3.4 Continuous data

Spatially continuous data such as rainfall, humidity, air pollution, or soil mineral concentrations may be estimated at all possible locations within a region of interest. The aim when dealing with continuous spatial variables is to collect data at a series of sampling locations and then to use that sample to estimate the value of the variable at other locations. Remotely sensed data are an exception to this statement as they provide complete coverage at the spatial resolution of the sensor. In epidemiology continuous variables of the type cited above may be used as covariates for predicting disease risk (see for example, Perry et al. (1991) and Hammond et al. (2001)).

Continuous spatial data are also used in transport models that investigate the distribution of agents released into the environment (Cromley and McLafferty 2002). These models require geographic and physical descriptions of the source, and information on the rate of release of the agent into the atmosphere, surface water, and/or land. Given the location of the source, and information on the

meteorology, hydrology, and hydrogeology of the environment into which an agent is released, the distribution of the agent throughout the environment can be predicted. A widely publicized application of fate and transport modelling applied in an epidemiological context was the *Escherichia coli* O157:H7 and *Campylobacter* outbreaks that occurred in the town of Walkerton, Ontario, Canada in May 2000 (Meyers et al. 2002). In this case, heavy rainfall resulted in bacteriological contamination of the town's water supply resulting in 2,300 clinical cases of gastrointestinal disease and seven deaths. Hydraulic modelling tools were used to trace contamination from the source to households within the affected area.

In the simplest situation, continuous data may be summarized by area unit and plotted as a choropleth map. This, however, ignores within-area variation of the variable of interest and, as with aggregated spatial data, large areas tend to dominate the map. Proportional symbol maps provide one solution to this problem where geometric symbols are plotted at each sampled location with the area of the symbol proportional to the value of the recorded value. Fig. 3.7 provides an example of this approach applied to the British cattle TB data. Circles of varying size have been used to indicate median herd size for each of the 178 areas shown in Fig. 3.3a. In Fig. 3.7 it is evident that herd sizes are largest in the east of the southwest region of England (label 'A'), Cheshire (label 'B'), and the Strathclyde region of Scotland (label 'C'). Linearly scaled symbols, such as bar charts, are an alternative to using geometric symbols and tend to be more accurately interpreted by map readers. A disadvantage of bar charts is that they become impractical when the range of data values plotted is large.

3.5 Effective data display

3.5.1 Media, scale, and area

When using fixed media such as paper, it is not possible to increase or decrease the scale of spatial resolution once a map has been prepared. GIS are much more flexible in this regard as 'zoom' facilities allow a map's resolution to be readily altered,

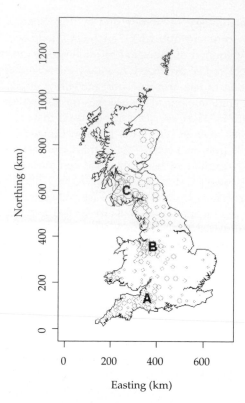

Figure 3.7 Proportional symbol map showing the spatial distribution of median cattle herd size throughout Great Britain. Key: A: the southwest of England, B: Cheshire, C: Strathclyde.

with greater spatial detail apparent at high levels of magnification and detail filtered from view at lower levels. Although this provides the cartographer with a great deal of flexibility it is important to be aware that the level of detail in the data at high resolutions is often not sufficient to support meaningful analysis. In some mapping applications (e.g. Google Earth[36]) additional data are automatically retrieved by the application when the user chooses to view the data at higher levels of spatial resolution.

In addition to issues related to resolution, care needs to be exercised when defining an area of study. In certain situations the area of interest may be clearly defined, for example, an entire country, island, or state. In other situations the definition of

---

[36] http://earth.google.com

the area of interest requires more care. For example, if the spatial distribution of disease around a possible pollution source is to be investigated, the distance over which the pollution source is expected to exert its influence needs to be considered. If the study area is too small it will be difficult to detect changes in disease density associated with distance from the source. Conversely, if the study area is too large then measures of disease prevalence summarized across the entire study area may fail to identify the presence of disease excess.

3.5.2 Dynamic display

An additional advantage of GIS over fixed media is that it is well suited for visualizing *dynamic* spatial patterns (i.e. where the spatial distribution of event information changes over time). Software protocols for data interchange such as Open Database Connectivity (ODBC) offer a means whereby a GIS can connect to a database 'on the fly' and extract information for display. This facility is of particular use in disease emergencies, where event information recorded into a central database can be displayed to users in real time.

Dynamic visualization can also be performed retrospectively. With retrospective analyses a series of maps can be created showing the spatial distribution of disease events identified within consecutive time frames. This map series can then be viewed in sequence allowing both the temporal and spatial distribution of the disease to be appreciated. This technique is particularly useful for communicating the results of analyses to a non-technical audience. Electronic formats are again useful in this regard as animated map projections can provide a 'movie' of how the spatial distribution of disease changes over time (see for example, Stevenson et al. (2000) and Thulke et al. (2000)). Fig. 3.8 provides a static example of this approach applied to the outbreak of foot-and-mouth disease (FMD) in the county of Cumbria, UK in 2001 (Wilesmith et al. 2003). Between February and March 2001 there was a relatively high density of disease incident cases in the northwest of the study area (Fig. 3.8a). For the period February to September the map series illustrates how the virus 'diffused' into the centre of the study area (Fig. 3.8b and Fig. 3.8c), and then

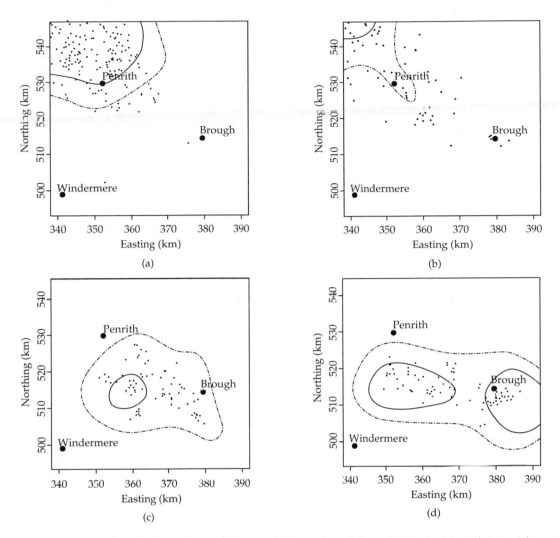

Figure 3.8 Contour plots illustrating the north-to-south 'movement' of foot-and-mouth disease (FMD) in Cumbria, UK between February and September 2001, where >10% (dashed lines) and >20% (solid lines) of holdings were diagnosed with FMD. (a) 20th February to 28th March, (b) 29th March to 23rd May, (c) 24th May to 18th July and (d) 19th July to 30th September. Point locations of incident holdings in each period have been superimposed for reference. Reproduced from Wilesmith et al. (2003) with permission from *Preventive Veterinary Medicine*.

moved in an east–west direction between July and September (Fig. 3.8d).

In a study of motor neurone disease in Finland, Sabel et al. (2000) acknowledge that the place of exposure to risk factors might not necessarily correspond to the place of physical emergence of disease as people move from one location to another throughout their lifetime. These authors use a three-dimensional approach to describe their data

(Fig. 3.9) which were collected using migration and health data registered on the personal level in Finland. It is expected that these types of analyses, linking space, time, and the movement of individuals through space and time will become more commonplace as systems are implemented routinely to record such detailed information and computer software and hardware become more powerful. In this sense a population is no longer

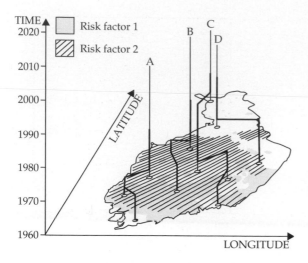

Figure 3.9 Three dimensional space–time prism. This figure demonstrates the changing life-paths for four individuals exposed to two risk factors in the geographic space of Finland. Reproduced from Sabel et al. (2000) with permission from *Social Science and Medicine.*

geographically defined since it encompasses people and animals at different locations, at different points in time.

3.5.3 Cartography

When developing a map, perhaps the first aspect that needs to be considered is the format that it will take. For example, a map developed for display on an internet web page will be quite different from a map used in a printed book or journal article. Maps intended for display on a computer screen can make use of colour and detailed symbols to identify features (if it is possible to pan and zoom), whereas printed maps within a book, journal, or thesis are often restricted to black and white and need to use simple symbology in order to identify features clearly.

Almost all maps should include basic details to provide the reader with key information about the data being mapped. These details include a map title, a scale, a legend, the body of the map (obviously), an indicator of north, and in some circumstances, the name of the cartographer, a neatline, the date of production, details of the map projection, and information about the source of data. Some of these elements are found on all maps while the presence of others depends on the context in which the map is placed. Scale bars, north arrows, legends, and source of information are required for all maps while neatlines, locator maps, and inset maps are elements that tend to be selectively used to further assist effective communication.

3.5.3.1 *Distance or scale*
As a rule of thumb, distance or scale should always be indicated on mapped data unless the intended audience is so familiar with the map's contents that the concept of distance can be assumed. There are two options for indicating distance or scale. Either a scale bar can be used, as in Fig. 3.10, or distance can be indicated as part of the labelling on the horizontal and vertical axes of the map, as in Fig. 3.8.

3.5.3.2 *Projection*
A projection transforms the area being mapped from the Earth's sphere to a flat page or screen. Projections necessarily distort the Earth so it is impossible in principle for the scale (i.e. distance on the map compared with distance on the Earth) of any flat map to be perfectly uniform, or the pixel size of any raster map to be perfectly constant. Projections can however preserve certain properties, the two most important being: (1) conformal property, which ensures that the shapes of small features are preserved on the projection (i.e. the scales of the projection in the x and y directions are always equal), and (2) equal area property, which ensures that areas measured on the map are always in the same proportion to areas on the Earth's surface. Conformal properties are important for

navigation while equal area properties are important for analyses involving areas.

Map projections can be divided into two groups, global and regional systems. Global projections (such as the Transverse Mercator projection and the Universal Transverse Mercator projection) are used to define position at all locations across the Earth's surface. Regional systems on the other hand are defined for specific areas, often covering countries, states or provinces. Typical examples are the British National Grid for Great Britain which is based on the Transverse Mercator projection, and the State Plane Coordinate System used in the United States. Projections that preserve area, such as regional systems, are most suitable for epidemiological mapping.

3.5.3.3 Direction
All maps should provide some indication of the direction of north. Similar to the depiction of distance, north can be depicted symbolically (as in Fig. 3.10) or can be inferred through the labelling of the horizontal and vertical axes. In Fig. 3.8 the title 'Northing' for the vertical axis indicates the direction of north. True north (the direction to the North Pole) differs from magnetic north, which changes due to changes in the characteristics of the condition of the Earth's crust and core. A map might indicate both true and magnetic north. If not, the convention is to indicate true north.

3.5.3.4 Legends
The map legend lists the symbols used on the map and what they depict. Symbols should appear in the legend exactly as they appear in the body of the map. Not all maps require a legend. Sometimes, particularly with simple maps, the required information can be included in the caption. In Fig. 3.8 the meaning of the dashed and solid contour lines is explained in the caption, primarily out of a need to provide an uncluttered display in each of the four maps that make up the series.

3.5.3.5 Neatlines, and locator and inset maps
Neatlines (also known as clipping lines) are used to frame a map and to indicate exactly where the area of the map begins and ends. Neatlines are also used to clip the body of the map and of locator or inset maps. Some maps may portray areas that are unfamiliar to readers and therefore, in order to provide readers with a better sense of the map context, a locator map is useful for showing where the mapped data is in relation to an area that is familiar to them. Sometimes mapped data are so densely clustered in small sections of a larger map that the cartographer must provide the reader with a close-up view of an area that is of specific interest. These detailed maps are called insets.

3.5.3.6 Symbology
Spatial attribute data can be classified as:

1. Nominal: attributes are nominal if they are given names or titles in order to distinguish one entity from another (e.g. place names).
2. Ordinal: attributes are ordinal if their values take on a natural order (e.g. agricultural land may be classed in terms of soil quality with Class 1 representing the best, Class 2 second-best, and so on).
3. Numeric: examples of numeric data include temperature, elevation, and rainfall. Numeric values may vary on a discrete (e.g. integer) or continuous scale.

Cartographers use symbols (points, lines, or areas) and combinations of shape, hue, orientation, size, and texture to communicate features of attribute data. The choice of graphic to depict spatial attribute data, and how best to position them on maps, are important considerations in optimizing map interpretability. The representation of nominal data by graphic symbols and icons is apparently trivial, although in practice automating placement to maximize clarity presents a range of analytical problems. Most GIS include generic algorithms for positioning labels and symbols around geographic objects. Point labels are positioned to avoid overlap by creating a window around text or symbols, linear features are labelled using splines, and area labels are assigned to central points, usually the centroid.

Ordinal attribute data are assigned to points, lines, and area objects in the same manner with the property of the data accommodated through the use of a hierarchy of graphic variables (symbol and lettering sizes, types, colours, intensities). Most users are unable to differentiate between more than seven ordinal categories and this provides an upper limit on the extent of the hierarchy.

A number of conventions are used when visualizing interval and ratio scale attribute data. Proportional circles and bar charts are often used to assign interval or ratio scale data to point or area locations, as in Fig. 3.7. Variable line width, with increments that correspond to the precision of the interval measure, is a standard convention for representing continuous variation in flow diagrams.

Variation in attribute data is usually represented by colour. Hue refers to the use of colour, principally to distinguish categories, for example in land use maps. Hues are usually ranked in order of lightness to reflect ordering in the data. The simplest approach is to use light to dark colours of a constant hue to represent low to high values, as in Fig. 3.2. Progression through adjacent hues, such as yellow–green–blue, makes it easier to accentuate differences between plotted symbols. Diverging data may have an obvious structure such as positive and negative values as in the case of residuals produced from a regression analysis (Chapter 7). Dark blue (for negative values) through white, to dark red (for positive values) is a useful colour scheme for representing this diverging structure.

About 8% of men and less than 1% of women have some form of colour blindness. Colour blind people are able to see many hues but there are predictable groupings of hues that are confused with each other, although the extent of this confusion depends on the severity of the person's colour vision deficiency. Hue pairs that work well for colour blind readers are red-blue, red-purple, orange-blue, yellow-blue, yellow-grey, and blue-grey. If spectral (rainbow) schemes are used, it is recommended to avoid the greens. A useful series of sequential colour schemes for mapping are provided by online sites such as ColorBrewer.[37] Tools are available for correcting the appearance of graphics for those with impaired colour vision.[38]

3.5.3.7 *Dealing with statistical generalization*
In spatial epidemiology maps are typically used to display statistical information. A common procedure is to show the spatial distribution of disease incidence, summarized by some level of administrative area. Maps prepared for this task need to depict, as accurately and as unambiguously as possible, the underlying distribution of the data. When mapping epidemiological data a balance needs to be struck between remaining true to the underlying data distribution and generalizing the data sufficiently to reveal the spatial pattern.

To illustrate this issue the British cattle TB data were used to produce a set of maps of holding-level prevalence of TB using different numbers of cut-points (Fig. 3.10). With small numbers of categories subtle features of the spatial distribution of disease are obscured (Fig. 3.10a). Similarly, too many categories are just as unproductive as large numbers of colours, and similarity of colour between adjacent areas, makes it difficult for the map-user to identify differences between adjacent areas (Fig. 3.10c). As a rule of thumb, it is difficult for most map-readers to distinguish more than about five to seven categories.

Six basic classification schemes have been developed to divide continuous attribute data into categories:

1. Natural breaks (Jenks method): Classes are defined according to apparently natural groupings of data values. The breaks may be defined by break points that are known to be relevant to a particular application, such as fractions and multiples of mean income levels, or rainfall thresholds known to support different levels of vegetation. Inductive classification of data values may be carried out whereby the GIS 'searches' for large jumps in data values.

2. Quantile breaks: Here the data are divided into a pre-determined number of classes which contain an equal number of observations. For example, quintile (five categories) classifications are well suited to displaying linearly distributed data.

3. Equal-interval breaks: This method takes the difference between the lowest and the highest attribute value and divides this difference into evenly spaced steps. Equal interval breaks are useful for mapping attribute data that follow a uniform distribution, or if the data ranges are familiar to the user of the map (e.g. herd sizes or temperature bands).

---

[37] http://www.colorbrewer.org
[38] http://www.vischeck.com

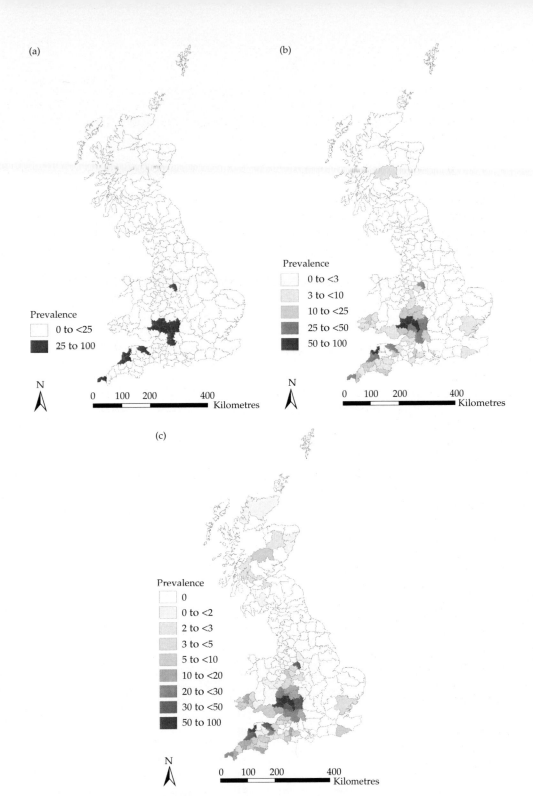

Figure 3.10 Choropleth maps showing area-level prevalence of TB on British cattle holdings (expressed as the number of TB-positive holdings per 100,000 holdings) for 1985–1997 plotted using (a) two, (b) five, and (c) nine cutpoints. See plate 4.

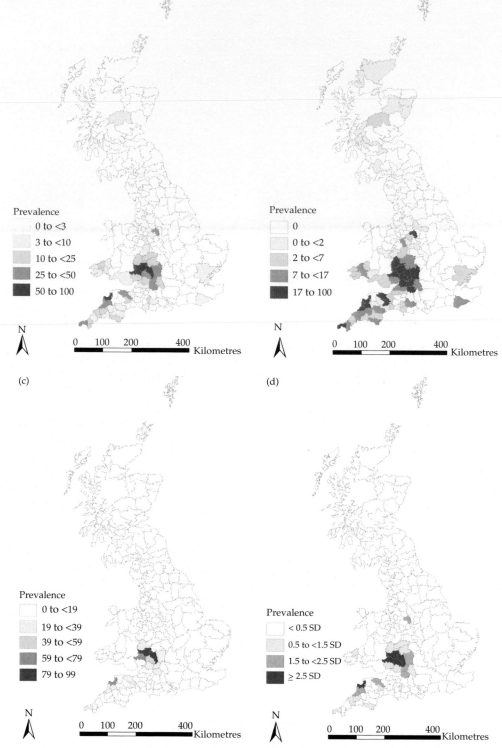

Figure 3.11 Choropleth maps showing area-level prevalence of TB on British cattle holdings (expressed as the number of TB-positive holdings per 100,000 holdings) for 1985–1997 using (a) natural breaks, (b) quintile breaks, (c) equal interval breaks, and (d) standard deviation classifications. See plate 5.

4. Standard deviation classifications: Here, the distance of the observation from the mean is shown. The GIS calculates the mean value and then generates class breaks in standard deviation measures above and below it. A two colour ramp helps to emphasize values above and below the mean. This method is most useful for attribute data that follow a normal distribution.

5. Arithmetic progressions: The widths of category intervals are increased in size at an arithmetic (additive) rate. For example, if the first category is one unit wide and it is decided to increment the width by one unit, the second category would be two units wide, the third three units wide, and so on (1, 3, 6, …). This method is particularly useful for skewed distributions.

6. Geometric progressions: The widths of the category intervals are increased in size at a geometric (multiplicative) rate. For example, if the first category is two units wide, the second category would be $2 \times 2 = 4$ units wide, the third category would be $2 \times 2 \times 2 = 8$ units wide, and so on (2, 6, 14…). Again, this method is particularly useful for skewed distributions.

In Fig. 3.11 the county-level prevalence of TB has been plotted using four to five categories, but the class breaks for each category were determined using natural breaks, quintile breaks, equal interval breaks, and standard deviation classifications.

Although these maps were all developed using the same dataset, they convey different spatial patterns to the user. Fig. 3.11b, for example, emphasizes the lower values in the distribution whereas Fig. 3.11c emphasizes the higher values. When choosing the number of classes to use, and an appropriate method to separate these classes, it helps to first plot the distribution of data values as a histogram. It is best to start with a standard classification and adjust the breaks to improve the map depending on the data and the target audience. If there are extreme outliers or large numbers of zero values, these can be placed into a class of their own, whilst the rest of the data can be classified using a standard method.

3.6 Conclusion

Disease maps play a key role in descriptive spatial epidemiology. Maps are useful for several purposes such as identification of areas with suspected elevations in risk, formulation of hypotheses about disease aetiology, and assessing needs for health-resource allocation. The production of attractive and informative maps complements the formal analysis of spatial epidemiological data, and as a result of the visual impact they have, it is likely that maps will influence the recipient much more than accompanying statistics (Rezaeian et al. 2004). As with any other form of data analysis, maps have the potential both to inform and to mislead. A key skill in spatial analysis therefore is 'to ensure that apparent geographical patterns are not artefacts of the mapping process' (Cliff 1995a). Investigators should, therefore, produce a variety of maps in order to illustrate particular aspects of their data and to validate the robustness of any inferences made (Gatrell and Bailey 1996). Choice of appropriate study area boundaries, distance and scale, geographic projection, symbology, linking maps with other forms of data display (e.g. dynamic spatial data analysis and conditioned choropleth maps), and dealing with statistical generalization are aspects of visualization that should be carefully considered in order to achieve these objectives.

CHAPTER 4

Spatial clustering of disease and global estimates of spatial clustering

4.1 Introduction

As described in Chapter 3, the ability to visualize spatial data allows for the quick identification of any obvious patterns, and in general, spatial patterns can be classified as regular, random, or clustered. The term 'clustering' is used to describe the spatial aggregation of disease events, but as the observed spatial pattern may simply be a function of the distribution of the population at risk or of various risk factors, a more robust definition is the one proposed by Wakefield et al. (2000), that a disease is clustered if there is 'residual spatial variation in risk after known influences have been accounted for'.

Besag and Newell (1991) classified the different methods for analysing clusters as either specific or non-specific, although epidemiologists prefer to use the terms 'local' and 'global'. Global (non-specific) clustering methods are used to assess whether clustering is apparent throughout the study region but do not identify the location of clusters. They provide a single statistic that measures the degree of spatial clustering, the statistical significance of which can then be assessed. The null hypothesis for global clustering methods is simply that 'no clustering exists' (i.e. random spatial dispersion). Local (specific) methods of cluster detection define the locations and extent of clusters, and can be further divided into focused and non-focused tests. Non-focused tests identify the location of all likely clusters in the study region, while focused tests investigate whether there is an increased risk of disease around a pre-determined point, such as a nuclear power plant or chemical factory. Bear in mind that the term *clustering* applies to global

methods of cluster analysis, while *cluster detection* refers to local methods of analysis.

Clustering of a disease can occur for a variety of reasons including the infectious spread of disease, the occurrence of disease vectors in specific locations, the clustering of a risk factor or combination of risk factors, or the existence of potential health hazards such as localized pollution sources scattered throughout a region, each creating an increased risk of disease in its immediate vicinity. The identification and reporting of areas with an apparent increased incidence of disease is known as a *disease cluster alarm*.

In this chapter a brief discussion of disease cluster alarms and cluster investigation protocols is followed by a review of some statistical concepts and terminology relevant to spatial clustering. The chapter concludes with an outline of some of the more commonly-used global clustering methods for point and area data, highlighting the advantages and disadvantages of each technique and exploring their application through a review of their use in the literature.

4.2 Disease cluster alarms and cluster investigation

The investigation of possible disease clustering is fundamental to epidemiology, with one of the aims being to determine whether the clustering is statistically significant and worthy of further investigation, or whether it is likely to be a chance occurrence, or is simply a reflection of the distribution of the population at risk. The statistical significance of clustering is especially important when studying the aetiology of a disease, when conducting disease surveillance programmes or when evaluating disease cluster alarms (Lawson and Kulldorff 1999). The false identification of a cluster in any of these situations may lead to wasted resources, while dismissing a genuine disease cluster can have serious consequences.

Although the reporting of suspected disease clusters is very common, only a minute proportion of these alarms are actually worthy of further investigation. Disease cluster alarms are usually based on a higher observed disease rate, a situation which can, understandably, cause concern among the public. By determining whether the observed clustering is *statistically* significant, disease cluster alarms can either be confirmed or rejected. In this way resources are not wasted on an in-depth assessment of what is frequently random spatial variation, yet at the same time scientific evidence is provided with which to allay public concern. As disease cluster alarms already define the extent of the cluster, thereby introducing pre-selection bias, it is not appropriate to determine the statistical significance of the cluster by simply comparing the standardized incidence or mortality rate within the cluster with that observed in the rest of the region. Statistical evaluation of the disease cluster alarm therefore has to take account of the pre-selection bias, and there are various ways in which this can be done. Either, the spatial scan statistic can be used to analyse data from the whole region in order to determine whether it identifies a significant cluster in the vicinity of the cluster alarm or, if the suspected cluster is the result of a potential health hazard (e.g. a landfill site), a focused cluster analysis (see Chapter 5) can be performed on the same health hazard but in a different area. A third approach is to ignore all prior data collected from the area of the alarm and instead, monitor any new cases that occur in the area. Kulldorff (1999) provides a detailed discussion of these three approaches, highlighting the strengths and weaknesses of each.

Investigating possible disease clusters requires a systematic approach and various cluster investigation protocols are available, details of which can be obtained from the EUROCAT website[39]. A widely

adopted method is the one outlined by the Centers for Disease Control and Prevention (CDC 1990), although Rothenberg and Thacker (1992) conclude that this protocol is not sufficiently specific to cover all possible eventualities. The EUROCAT Working Group recommends the Dutch Triple Track approach (Drijver and Melse 1992) for investigating clusters as this protocol proposes simultaneously investigating the health effects and environmental exposures, while communicating with the public, rather than following the sequential approach frequently adopted by other protocols. For instance, the first step (orientation) of the Dutch Triple Track approach to disease cluster investigation requires the collection of general information on the expected disease frequency and potential risk factors (health track), and on local exposure possibilities (environment track), while preparing a visit to the person who contacted the health agency (communication track).

4.3 Statistical concepts relevant to cluster analysis

4.3.1 Stationarity, isotropy, and first- and second-order effects

The concepts of stationarity, isotropy, and first-order (trend) and second-order (local) spatial effects are introduced in Chapter 2, and are fundamental to cluster analysis. To summarize, a spatial process is termed stationary if the dependence between measurements of the same variable across space is the same for all locations in an area. If the dependence in a stationary process is affected by distance, but this is the same in all directions, the process is considered to be isotropic. First-order effects describe large-scale variations in the mean of the outcome of interest due to location or other explanatory variables, while second-order effects describe small-scale variation due to interactions between neighbours.

4.3.2 Monte Carlo simulation

Many tests for clustering use Monte Carlo simulation in order to determine the statistical significance of the cluster (i.e. does the observed spatial

---

[39] http://www.eurocat.ulster.ac.uk/clusterinvprot.html

pattern differ significantly from the null hypothesis of complete spatial randomness). This involves first calculating the test statistic using the *observed* data, and then re-calculating it using a specified number (e.g. 99, 499, 999) of *simulated* data sets (or permutations). The latter is used to generate the expected distribution of the test statistic under the null hypothesis. The likelihood of obtaining the value for the test statistic derived from the observed data is then calculated, and expressed as the p-value. A Monte Carlo estimate of the p-value for a one-sided test is given by the proportion of test statistic values, obtained from the simulated datasets, that are greater than the value of the test statistic obtained when using the observed data. As Monte Carlo methods rely on permutations of simulated datasets, slightly different p-values are obtained each time the test is run. However, using more simulations to estimate the distribution of the null hypothesis (e.g. 999 versus 99), means that smaller and more stable p-values can be calculated (e.g. $p = 0.001$ as opposed to $p = 0.01$). However, a problem with multiple testing is that the likelihood of wrongly rejecting the null hypothesis increases. To compensate the significance threshold needs to be lowered and this is usually done using either a Bonferroni or Simes adjustment.

4.3.3 Statistical power of clustering methods

This chapter discusses some of the more commonly-used cluster analysis methods, and although certain tests are more appropriately used in specific situations, when there are competing methods a commonly asked question is 'which is best'? In such instances, the statistical power of the test (i.e. the probability of detecting clustering or clusters when they actually occur) can provide an answer. Waller and Gotway (2004) discuss various issues affecting the ability of a test to correctly detect clustering, including the structure of the data and the alternative hypothesis. A comparison of the performance of different clustering methods is provided in Walter (1992; 1993), Kulldorff et al. (2003), Song and Kulldorff (2003) and Kulldorff et al. (2006a). When compared with other global clustering tests, Tango's maximized excess events test (MEET) has been found to be the most consistent

for evaluating cancer maps (Kulldorff et al. 2006a) and have the highest power of the tests under evaluation (Kulldorff et al. 2003; Song and Kulldorff 2003). Cuzick and Edwards' k-nearest neighbour test has also been shown to perform well, especially when the clustering occurrs over small distances (Kulldorff et al. 2003). A detailed discussion of the statistical power of clustering and cluster detection methods can be found in Waller and Gotway (2004).

4.4 Methods for aggregated data

Autocorrelation statistics for aggregated data provide an estimate of the degree of spatial similarity observed among neighbouring values of an attribute over a study area. There are various autocorrelation statistics for aggregated data, four of which will be discussed in this section; Moran's I, Geary's c; Tango's excess events test and maximized excess events test. Details of other autocorrelation tests can be found in Cliff and Ord (1973; 1981).

Fundamental to all autocorrelation statistics is the weights matrix, used to define the spatial relationships of the regions so that those that are close in space are given greater weight in the calculation than those that are distant (Moran 1950). Neighbours can be defined based either on adjacency or distance. Methods based on adjacency (also known as contiguity) include rook contiguity (polygons are adjacent if they share a border), queen contiguity (polygons are adjacent if they share a border or corner), and higher-order contiguities (often called spatial lags) such as first-order (neighbours) or second-order adjacency (neighbours-of-neighbours). The concept of higher-order adjacencies is illustrated in Fig. 4.1. When using distance to define neighbours, polygons with their centroids located within a specified distance range are considered to be adjacent. More complicated neighbour definitions include row-standardization, length of common boundary, or relationships that only act one way (e.g. large polygons may influence, but not be influenced by, neighbouring, smaller polygons). Software for producing the weights matrix includes GeoDa and ArcView.

(a) (b)

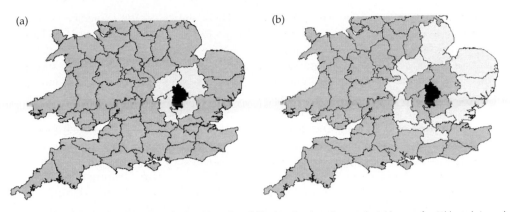

Figure 4.1 Maps illustrating (a) first-order adjacency (neighbours), and (b) second-order adjacency (neighbours-of-neighbours). In each instance the black county is the polygon of interest and the light-grey counties the defined neighbours.

4.4.1 Moran's *I*

Moran's *I* coefficient of autocorrelation is similar to Pearson's correlation coefficient, and quantifies the similarity of an outcome variable among areas that are defined as spatially related (Moran 1950). Moran's *I* statistic is given by:

$$I = \frac{n\sum_i\sum_j W_{ij}(Z_i - \overline{Z})(Z_j - \overline{Z})}{(\sum_i\sum_j W_{ij})\sum_k(Z_k - \overline{Z})^2} \qquad (4.1)$$

where Z_i could be the residuals $(O_i - E_i)$ or standardized mortality or morbidity ratio (SMR) of an area, and W_{ij} is a measure of the closeness of areas *i* and *j*. A weights matrix is used to define the spatial relationships so that regions close in space are given greater weight when calculating the statistic than those that are distant (Moran 1950).

Moran's *I* is approximately normally distributed and has an expected value of $-1/(N - 1)$ (where *N* equals the number of area units within a study region), when no correlation exists between neighbouring values. The expected value of the coefficient therefore approaches zero as *N* increases. Although Moran's *I* generally lies between +1 and -1, it is not bound by these limits (unlike Pearson's correlation coefficient; Waller and Gotway 2004). A Moran's *I* of zero indicates the null hypothesis of no clustering, a positive Moran's *I* indicates positive spatial autocorrelation (i.e. clustering of areas of similar attribute values), while a negative coefficient indicates

negative spatial autocorrelation (i.e. that neighbouring areas tend to have dissimilar attribute values). The significance of Moran's *I* can be assessed using Monte Carlo randomization (Moran 1950). Moran's *I* can be calculated using various software packages, including ClusterSeer, R, and GeoDa.

Disadvantages of the autocorrelation test are the assumptions that the population at risk is evenly distributed within the study area (Moran 1950), and that the correlation or covariance is the same in all directions (i.e. it is isotropic). The problems posed by anisotropic data can be overcome by manipulating the weights matrix to reflect directional inequalities.

Although Moran's *I* is intended for use with continuous data it can also be used to analyse count data, even though, in such instances, any observed autocorrelation may simply be the result of variation in regional population sizes rather than any genuine spatial pattern in the disease counts (e.g. if regions with large populations are grouped together). Accounting for the population at risk by using regional incidence rates, instead of regional disease counts, increases the likelihood that any observed autocorrelation reflects a genuine spatial pattern rather than a heterogeneous population distribution.

A spatial correlogram is a series of estimates of Moran's *I* evaluated at increasing distances. Moran's *I* is plotted on the vertical axis and distance (spatial lag) is plotted on the horizontal axis.

The correlogram can therefore be used to determine where, on average, spatial autocorrelation is maximized. Correlograms can be calculated based on distance or adjacency. There are various tests to determine whether a spatial autocorrelation value in a correlogram is statistically significant, some of which are reviewed by Cliff and Ord (1981). A correlogram differs from a semivariogram (described in Chapter 6) in that the former plots correlation against distance, while the latter plots the semivariance against distance (correlation being a measure of the similarity, and semivariance a measure of the dissimilarity, between the variable under consideration and the lagged version of the same variable).

As Moran's I cannot adjust for a heterogeneous population density, Oden (1995) proposed the use of Oden's $Ipop$, a test statistic similar to Moran's I but in which rates are adjusted for population size.

In the following example, Moran's I was used to test whether there was clustering of counties in Great Britain in 1999 with respect to TB incidence rates. Using the GeoDA software, a weights matrix based on queen contiguity (i.e. polygons having a common border or corner) and a spatial lag of one (i.e. first-order adjacency) was defined and used in conjunction with Monte Carlo randomization (999 permutations), to calculate Moran's I for the data.

These indicated the existence of non-significant, ($p = 0.085$) positive, spatial autocorrelation ($I = 0.0832$) in the TB incidence rates of neighbouring counties. In order to investigate spatial autocorrelation at higher-order spatial lags, weights matrices were defined and Moran's I statistics calculated for second- to fourth-order adjacencies, and used to plot a correlogram (Fig. 4.2), which illustrates that for first- and second-order adjacencies spatial autocorrelation was positive, but negative for higher-order adjacencies. In other words, neighbouring or nearly-neighbouring counties (spatial lag of one or two) had similar TB incidence rates (either high or low), whereas counties further away from the one of interest (spatial lag of three or four) tended to have dissimilar incidence rates.

There are many examples of the use of Moran's I in the literature. Kitron and Kazmierczak (1997) use Moran's I to investigate the spatial distribution of the incidence of Lyme disease by county, between 1991 and 1994 in Wisconsin State, USA, and analyse clustering in two candidate covariates of Lyme disease; the distribution of the tick vector *Ixodes scapularis* and Normalized Difference Vegetation Index (NDVI) values, derived from the National Oceanic and Atmospheric Administration's (NOAA) Advanced Very High Resolution Radiometer

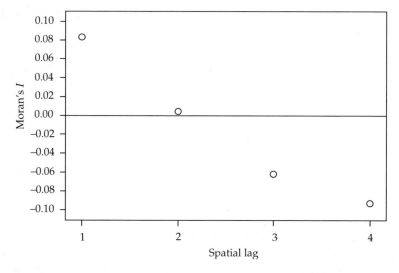

Figure 4.2 A correlogram showing Moran's I statistic computed for TB incidence rates in Great Britain in 1999 at first, second, third, and fourth-order spatial lags.

(AVHRR), during spring and autumn when the contrast between agricultural land and woodland is maximized. Assigning data for each county to its centroid, they calculate Moran's I statistic and use spatial correlograms to evaluate the distances where spatial effects are greatest. This analysis demonstrates significant clustering of counties for mean annual incidence of Lyme disease, tick endemicity, and NDVI values in spring and autumn.

Moran's I is also used by Bellec et al. (2006) to investigate spatial autocorrelation of cases of childhood acute leukaemia in France between 1990 and 2000, and by Perez et al. (2002) to investigate clustering of bovine TB in Argentina. Nødtvedt et al. (2007) use Moran's I to assess autocorrelation of incidence rates of canine atopic dermatitis in Sweden.

4.4.2 Geary's c

Geary's contiguity ratio, or Geary's c, is another weighted estimate of spatial autocorrelation (Geary 1954) but whereas Moran's I considers similarity between neighbouring regions, Geary's c considers similarity between *pairs* of regions. Geary's c ranges from zero to two, with zero indicating perfect positive spatial autocorrelation and two indicating perfect negative spatial autocorrelation, for any pair of regions. Geary's c is given by:

$$c = \frac{(n-1)\sum_{i=1}^{n}\sum_{j=1}^{n}w_{ij}(y_i - y_j)^2}{2\left(\sum_{i=1}^{n}(y_i - \bar{y})^2\right)\left(\sum_{i=1}^{n}\sum_{j=1}^{n}w_{ij}\right)} \qquad (4.2)$$

where n is the number of polygons in the study area, w_{ij} the values of the spatial proximity matrix, y_i the attribute under investigation, and the mean of the attribute under investigation.

4.4.3 Tango's excess events test (EET) and maximized excess events test (MEET)

Tango (1995) developed the excess events test (EET) to measure the 'closeness' among regions based on a distance matrix. Tango's EET is a weighted sum of excess events, as the statistic considers the difference between the observed rate of cases in each region and the expected rate, and then weights

these differences by a measure of the distance between the regions, with a higher weighting given when the two locations are close.

Unfortunately Tango's EET requires the parameter λ (a measure of the spatial scale of clustering) to be specified, resulting in two problems. Firstly, λ is not generally known *a priori* and therefore several values of λ are tested creating issues of multiple testing. Secondly, choosing a large λ makes the test sensitive to geographically large-scale clustering while a small λ makes it more sensitive to small-scale clustering. To overcome these problems, Tango (2000) proposed the maximized excess events test (MEET). This test statistic searches for the value of λ which gives the smallest p-value of the observed value of the test statistic.

The MEET performs well using the two distance-based exponential weight functions proposed by Tango (2000). However, Song and Kulldorff (2005) evaluate other potential weight functions, concluding that the power of the test improves when using functions that incorporate information on the spatial relationship between areas compared to functions that do not. For example, the weight may be defined purely by Euclidean distance or in terms of spatial contiguity of regions, or it could be adjusted according to population density so that the weight declines faster in urban than in rural areas (Song and Kulldorff 2005).

There are few examples of Tango's EET or MEET in the literature. Fang et al. (2004) use Tango's EET to identify significant clustering of brain cancer mortality rates among adults in the United States between 1986 and 1995, while Oliver et al. (2006) use Tango's MEET to identify significant clustering of prostate cancer incidence in Virginia between 1990 and 1999.

4.5 Methods for point data

4.5.1 Cuzick and Edwards' k-nearest neighbour test

Cuzick and Edwards (1990) developed a test for spatial clustering that takes into account the potentially heterogeneous distribution of the population at risk. It is based on the locations of cases and randomly selected controls from a specified region and includes a spatial scale parameter k, determined by the user. Scale in this instance refers to the number of nearest neighbours, and not geographic distance. For each case, the test counts how many of the k-nearest neighbours are also cases, such that if there are n_1 cases, and $m_i(k)$ represents the number of cases among the k nearest neighbours of case i so that $0 \leq m_i(k) \leq k$, for $i = 1, \ldots n_1$, a test statistic T_k can be calculated as follows:

$$T_k = \sum_{i=1}^{n_1} m_i(k) \qquad (4.3)$$

Thus, when cases are clustered, the nearest neighbour to a case tends to be another case and T_k will be large. However, when all cases have controls as their nearest neighbours T_k will be zero. The observed value of T_k can be compared with the distribution of values computed using Monte Carlo randomization of the dataset (Wakefield et al. 2000).

When data are available for the population at risk a modification of T_k is:

$$U_k = \sum_{j=1}^{n_1} (Y_j - E_j) \qquad (4.4)$$

where circular regions are centred on each case and the radius of each circular region is chosen so that the expected number cases, E_j, is as close to the pre-defined value of k as possible, and Y_j is the number of cases within each region. Under the null hypothesis the expected value of U_k is equal to zero and the variance may be calculated (Cuzick and Edwards 1990). The Cuzick and Edwards test can be implemented using the ClusterSeer software.

Information on the exact locations of cases and controls is not always available, with locations instead being frequently assigned to the centre of administrative areas such as counties or parishes. As a result of assigning cases and controls to the same area 'ties' arise, precluding the calculation of Cuzick and Edwards' test statistic. Jacquez (1994) proposed an extension to Cuzick and Edwards' method that allows the test to be used in such situations.

A distinct advantage of Cuzick and Edwards' method is that it takes account of the heterogeneous distribution of the population at risk, as cases and controls are selected from the same population. In this way, the existence of any clustering of the population at risk, such as in built-up areas is accounted for. Furthermore, through the careful selection of controls, this method allows confounders to be accounted for (Jacquez 1994). Disadvantages of the test include the fact that the user is required to select a value for the parameter k (Kulldorff et al. 2006a), and that interval data must be categorized as 'case' and 'control' locations resulting in a possible loss of information, although at the same time, this aspect of the test allows for flexibility in defining case and control locations (Ward and Carpenter 2000). For instance, cases may be locations where disease has been detected or alternately, locations at which disease is above a specified threshold, such as the mean disease prevalence (Ward and Carpenter 1995). Although Cuzick and Edwards' test was originally developed for use with point data it can easily be adapted for aggregated data (Song and Kulldorff 2003). When the unit of analysis is aggregated, defining cases and controls can require careful thought in order to avoid the introduction of bias.

Cuzick and Edwards (1990) apply this cluster detection method to explore the distribution of childhood leukaemia and lymphoma diagnosed in North Humberside between 1974 and 1986, an example that highlights the importance of selecting a suitable value of k, as the authors point out that 'formal significance testing requires either foreknowledge of the best k or some adjustment for multiple testing', such as a Bonferroni or Simes p-value adjustment.

There are many examples of Cuzick and Edwards test in the literature. Carpenter et al. (2006), using the Cuzick and Edwards method with multiple definitions for cases, find no evidence of spatial clustering of abortions among Danish dairy herds. Doherr et al. (2002) use the test to identify geographical clustering of BSE in Switzerland in animals born after imposition of the feed ban of December 1990. Perez et al. (2002) investigate clustering of bovine TB in Argentina, for which data are aggregated by county. Counties with a prevalence greater than the median are defined as cases, and those with a prevalence lower than or equal to the median as controls. Overall significance of clustering is assessed using values of k ranging from one to 10. Although no significant overall clustering is detected, significant clustering of case counties is detected at $k=1$ and $k=2$ suggesting that clustering of TB in Argentina is present at a relatively small spatial scale, with an elevated likelihood of disease occurrence only in neighbouring, or nearly neighbouring case counties.

4.5.2 Ripley's *K*-function

Second-order analysis describes the spatial dependence between events of the same type. The *K*-function is the most commonly-used method and identifies the distance at which clustering occurs. For an isotropic process with an intensity of λ points per unit area, the *K*-function at distance s may be defined as $K(s)$ such that $\lambda K(s)$ gives the expected number of events within a distance s of an arbitrarily-chosen event. Formally, $K(s)$ is defined as:

$$K(s) = \frac{1}{\lambda^2 R} \sum_{i \neq j} \sum I_s(d_{ij})$$ (4.5)

where R equals the area of a region of interest, d_{ij} is the distance between the ith and jth events in R, and $I_s(d_{ij})$ is an indicator function which equals 1 if $d_{ij} \leq s$ and 0 otherwise. Where spatial autocorrelation is present, each event is likely to be in close proximity to other members of the same event type and, for small values of s, $K(s)$ will be large.

An important assumption of the *K*-function is that there are no first-order effects in the spatial pattern, as any evidence of spatial trend may influence the computed *K*-function. In addition, the variance of $K(s)$ increases with increasing distance, and therefore the *K*-function is suitable for estimating general tendencies toward clustering over distances that are small compared with the size of the region (Diggle 2003). As a rule of thumb it is recommended to restrict the range of s to no greater than 0.5 times the length of the shorter side of a rectangular study area.

Due to variations in the spatial distribution of the population at risk, a *K*-function computed only for cases may not be very informative. Instead, the *K*-function calculated for cases ($K_{case}(s)$) can be compared with one calculated for non-cases (or

controls) ($K_{control}(s)$), with the difference between the two functions,

$$D(S) = K_{case}(s) - K_{control}(s)$$ (4.6)

representing a measure of the extra aggregation of cases over and above that observed for the non cases (Diggle and Chetwynd 1991). Monte Carlo randomization can then be used to randomly permute the locations of cases and non-cases/controls, and values of the difference function $D(s)$ computed for each permutation (Chetwynd and Diggle 1998). The upper and lower bounds of these permutations are then plotted together with the observed difference function $D(s)$. Any deviation of $D(s)$ above the envelope formed by the upper and lower bounds indicates significant clustering of cases, relative to non-cases/controls. The software for calculating the *K*-function includes ClusterSeer, or the splancs package (Rowlingson and Diggle 1993) adapted for use in R.

Advantages of using the *K*-function to investigate clustering include the fact that it does not depend on the shape of the study region, and precise spatial locations of events are used in its estimation (Cressie 1993). It also takes into account the density of events in the region of interest, enabling spatial dependence to be compared among groups regardless of event prevalence (Diggle 2003; Broman et al. 2006). Furthermore, the test can accommodate an edge-correction weighting factor, the most commonly used of which was proposed by Ripley (1976), although other edge-correction strategies can be found in Ripley (1988), Stoyan et al. (1995), Diggle (2003), and Waller and Gotway (2004).

In the following example of spatial clustering, the British cattle TB data were used to determine the distance over which clustering of TB-positive holdings was significant in a 60×60 km^2 area in the north-east of Cornwall in 1999. The analysis was performed using the splancs package in R. The TB-status of all holdings in this area is shown in Fig. 4.3a. *K*-functions were plotted for the TB-positive holdings (Fig. 4.3b) and for all the holdings (Fig. 4.3c) in the area of interest. Monte Carlo randomization was then used to randomly permute the locations of cases and non-cases, and values of the difference function ($D(s)$) computed for each permutation. The upper and lower bounds of these permutations were then plotted together with the observed difference function $D(s)$ (Fig. 4.3d). As described above, any deviation of $D(s)$ above the envelope formed by the upper and lower bounds indicates significant clustering of cases, relative to non-cases. In other words, compared with the spatial distribution of the holding population at risk, TB-positive holdings showed a greater tendency to be aggregated at distances of between 2 and 30 km, with maximum clustering occurring at a distance of 17 km.

O' Brien et al. (2000) use the K-function to investigate clustering of different types of neoplasms in humans and dogs in Michigan, USA between 1964 and 1994, concluding that the processes determining spatial aggregation of cases in the two species are not independent of one another. Abernethy et al. (2000) use the K-function to identify spatial clustering of poultry flocks affected with Newcastle disease in Northern Ireland between 1996 and 1997.

Broman et al. (2006) apply the K-function to investigate the effect of treatment on the clustering of ocular chlamydial infection in children among households in a Tanzanian village. Initially, clustering of households with high levels of infection occurs at distances of less than 2 km, suggesting

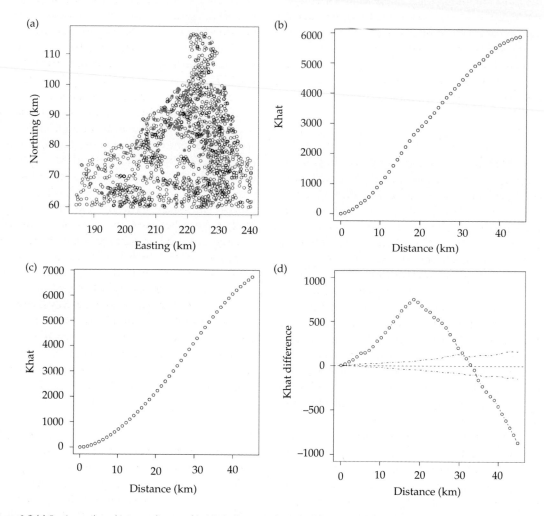

Figure 4.3 (a) Easting and northing coordinates of holdings that tested positive (•) and negative (○) for TB in a 60 × 60 km² area of Cornwall, (b) K-function for TB-positive holdings, (c) K-function for all holdings, and (d) the difference between the two K-functions.

that either the spread of infection occurs on a relatively small spatial scale or that nearby households share common risk factors for infection. Two months after treatment clustering is no longer evident, but by 12 months post-treatment clustering of households with high infection levels is again apparent, at distances of less than 1.3 km, indicating that treatment was effective at disrupting the spread of infection but not at maintaining low levels of the disease.

4.5.3 Rogerson's cumulative sum (CUSUM) method

Rogerson (1997) developed a cumulative sum (CUSUM) statistic for detecting changes in spatial pattern using a modified version of Tango's statistic (Tango 1995). Whereas Tango's test is used retrospectively to identify clustering, Rogerson's modified version of the statistic aims to detect emerging clusters shortly after they occur, and can therefore be used for spatial surveillance. Owing to the problem of multiple testing, it would be inappropriate simply to re-calculate Tango's statistic after each new observation. Instead, once the test statistic has been determined for a particular set of observations, the expected value and variance of Tango's statistic after the next observation is estimated, based on the current value of the statistic. The expected value and variance is then used to convert the Tango's statistic that is observed after the next observation into a z-score, with all z-scores being incorporated into a CUSUM framework (Rogerson 2006). As Rogerson's CUSUM method is based on Tango's statistic, the test includes a measure of the spatial scale of clustering (λ) and thus, choosing a small value of λ makes the test more sensitive to small clusters and *vice versa*. Although Rogerson (1997) chose to base his CUSUM method on Tango's statistic he suggests that similar CUSUM statistics can be developed for other measures of spatial pattern. For example, Moran's I could be used for aggregated data, or Cuzick and Edwards' method for point data. Rogerson's CUSUM method can be implemented using the ClusterSeer software.

Rogerson (1997) uses his CUSUM version of Tango's test to investigate clustering of cases of Burkitt's lymphoma in Uganda between 1961 and 1975, and finds that spatial clustering exists in specific time-intervals, thereby corroborating the findings of Williams et al. (1978) who had previously obtained similar results analysing the data using the chi-squared test and the Knox test for space–time interaction.

4.6 Investigating space–time clustering

While spatial patterns of disease are of great interest, space–time interactions are also important, particularly so when trying to determine whether a disease is infectious. In such instances it is necessary to evaluate whether cases that are close in space are also close in time and *vice versa*, adjusting for any purely spatial or temporal clustering. Various tests have been developed for this purpose; the tests for global space–time clustering are briefly reviewed in this chapter, while the local space–time cluster detection tests are dealt with in Chapter 5. It is worth noting that some tests look for clusters that relate to a fixed point in space, whilst others allow the spatial focus to move with time. In the first instance, the idea of a two-dimensional circular scan window is extended to that of a cylinder passing through time. In the second case, the geographical focus of a cluster may migrate with time, as long as it relates back to previous events. There is also an important distinction between tests that require knowledge of the population at risk, and those that do not. Not requiring population or control data has obvious advantages in terms of ease of implementation, but has a serious drawback in that it assumes that any change in the population at risk occurs evenly across the distribution under study (Kulldorff 1988). This would obviously have serious analytical implications, where interventions such as culling or vaccination may cause highly inhomogeneous changes in the population at risk.

4.6.1 The Knox test

Knox and Bartlett (1964) developed the first technique to identify spatio-temporal clustering of disease events and, although it has been the subject of much criticism, Knox's test has formed the platform from which subsequent tests have been developed. In this method, pairs of cases separated by less than a user-defined critical space-distance are considered to be near in space, and pairs of cases separated by less than a user-defined critical time-distance are said to be near in time. This classification allows pairs of points to be assigned to one of four cells in a 2 × 2 contingency table (near space – near time, near space – far time, far space – near time, far space – far time), and a test statistic, T_K is calculated as the number of pairs of cases that are near to one another in both space and time. The test statistic is compared against simulated results under a Poisson model, which Knox argues is the sampling distribution of the statistic in the absence of space-time clustering. Knox and Bartlett (1964) apply this method to data on cases of childhood leukaemia in northeast England, finding significant evidence of space–time clustering.

Jacquez (1996) highlights two principal limitations with Knox's test. Firstly, that the choice of critical distances is subjective and secondly, that the critical distance in space does not vary with changing population density. This is unrealistic since the distance from case to case would decrease with increasing population density. Baker (1996) discusses the problems associated with specifying thresholds of proximity in space and time in the Knox test, and develops an adaptation that does not require unknown critical parameters to be specified, but instead allows for a range to be given for each. In its most flexible form the range can be specified from zero to the maximum space and time differences between any two pairs of cases. The test becomes more powerful as the ranges for thresholds can be specified with increasing accuracy, and reduces to the Knox test itself when the range for each parameter is reduced to zero. He compares this test with a number of examples to which the Knox test had been applied. In the first instance, an exploration of cardiac defects among newborns identifies non-significant space–time clustering, compared with a significant result from the standard Knox test. In the second instance, involving Kaposi's sarcoma in the West Nile district of Uganda, the standard Knox test produces non-significant results whilst re-analysis with Baker's adaptation (Baker 1996) suggests the existence of space–time clustering.

Kulldorff and Hjalmars (1999) review the Knox method, and discuss in some detail its statistical

limitations, such as the problems of population-shift bias and the subjective choice of critical thresholds. They propose a modification of the test that overcomes these problems which they demonstrate using cases of lung cancer in New Mexico (1973–1991). Using the standard Knox test, significant space–time clustering is indicated at a range of critical distances whilst with their adaptation it is not. They show that changes in the distribution of the population at risk over time can have a strong influence on the standard test. These effects are particularly interesting with animal diseases where populations may be culled.

More recent applications of the Knox method include Norström et al. (2000), who investigate outbreaks of acute respiratory disease in Norwegian cattle herds, and Tinline et al. (2002), who use the method to estimate the incubation period of racoon rabies.

4.6.2 The space–time *k*-function

Diggle et al. (1995) extend existing second-order analysis methods for spatial data (Ripley 1976; 1977) in order to investigate space–time interactions in point process data. They find second-order properties to be closely related to Knox's statistic (Knox and Bartlett 1964), of which they refer to their test as an extension. If $K_S(s)$ defines the K-function in space and $K_T(t)$ defines the K-function in time, the K-function difference $D(s,t)$ is:

$$D(s,t) = K(s,t) - K_S(s)K_T(t) \qquad (4.7)$$

$D(s,t)$ estimates the cumulative number of cases expected within distance s and time-interval t of an arbitrarily-selected case attributable to the interaction between space and time. An alternative expression is:

$$D_0(s,t) = \frac{D(s,t)}{K_S(s)K_T(t)} \qquad (4.8)$$

which estimates, for given distance and time separations, the proportional increase in cases attributable to space–time interaction (Diggle et al. 1995).

French et al. (1999) apply the space–time K-function to investigate sheep scab outbreaks in Great Britain (1973–1992), revealing strong evidence that disease occurrence is clustered in both space and time. Wilesmith et al. (2003) and Picardo et al. (2007) both use the space–time K-function to investigate different aspects of the 2001 UK FMD epidemic. French et al. (2005) find strong evidence for space–time clustering of equine grass sickness cases using the space–time K-function, and suggest that this may be attributable either to a contagious process or to other spatially and temporally localized processes, such as pasture management practices or local climatic effects. Porphyre et al. (2007) use the space–time K-function to investigate whether the persistence of TB in a region of New Zealand is the result of contact between infected farms and conclude that there is no evidence of an increased TB risk for those farms close in time and space to TB-positive farms. Software for implementing the space–time K-function includes the splancs package in R.

4.6.3 The Ederer–Myers–Mantel (EMM) test

Ederer et al. (1964) developed a cell occupancy approach for exploring space–time clustering whereby the study region is divided into a series of space–time sub-regions within which unusual distributions of cases are sought. They demonstrate the Ederer–Myers–Mantel (EMM) test, using data on cases of childhood leukaemia in Connecticut (1945–1959) and find no evidence of space–time clustering, in contrast to data on poliomyelitis (1940–1954) and infectious hepatitis (1953–1962), both of which did show strong evidence for clustering in space and time. Fosgate et al. (2002) apply the EMM test to evaluate clustering of human brucellosis in California (1973–1977), finding significant space–time clustering that they attribute to clustering of work or food-related disease risk factors.

4.6.4 Mantel's test

Mantel (1967) reviews the methods of Knox and Bartlett (1964) and Ederer et al. (1964), and proposes a new test that compares inter-event distances in space and time against a null hypothesis that time and space distances are independent. The test statistic T_M is the sum, across all pairs of cases, of the spatial distances multiplied by the time distances.

A transformation is used to reduce the effects of large space and time distances, which would not be expected to be correlated for contagious diseases. Significance levels are then tested using a standard Monte Carlo randomization process.

Jacquez (1996) highlights a number of limitations of Mantel's test, in particular the linear form of the statistic. For most disease processes a non-linear relationship would be expected between space and time distances. Whilst this can be accounted for by transforming the data, the choice of transformation is subjective.

Wartenberg and Greenberg (1990) compare the statistical power of the tests developed by Ederer et al. (1964) and by Mantel (1967). They suggest that both tests have low statistical power for the typically small numbers of cases involved in such studies, and conclude that true clinical disease excesses, as might result from proximity to a single pollution source, are more likely to be detected by the EMM method whilst the Mantel method is more likely to detect hotspots such as those due to a more general exposure to a putative source.

4.6.5 Barton's test

Barton et al. (1965) designed a test to detect changes in spatial patterns associated with the passage of time, based on analysis of variance and which tests the null hypothesis that these patterns do not change with time. They illustrate their test using three datasets and, although unable to demonstrate significant space–time clustering of cases of childhood leukaemia in northeast England, for which Knox and Bartlett (1964) had previously found evidence of space–time clustering, they did identify space–time associations for measles in Southall in 1954, and poliomyelitis in Eccles in 1974. Ekstrand and Carpenter (1998) use Barton's test to demonstrate significant space–time clustering of flocks with very high prevalence of foot-pad dermatitis in Swedish broilers.

4.6.6 Jacquez's k nearest neighbours test

Jacquez (1996) developed a k nearest neighbours test for space–time interaction. The null hypothesis is of no association between time and space adjacencies (i.e. that the probability of two events being nearest neighbours in space is independent of the probability of their being nearest neighbours in time). This approach is based on the argument that geographic distance is not a good measure of spatial proximity in an epidemiological context. Jacquez (1996) compares the statistical power of his test against those of Knox and Mantel using a computer simulation of a viral epidemic at a range of cluster sizes. By plotting statistical power against cluster size he shows that the k nearest neighbours test performs considerably better than the other two, of which Mantel's test was superior. He also proposes an adaptation of the k nearest neighbours test using fuzzy set theory to accommodate imprecision in the spatial and temporal nearest neighbours.

Norström et al. (2000) compare Jacquez's k nearest neighbours to the Knox test in an investigation of outbreaks of acute respiratory disease in Norwegian cattle herds. They find strong evidence of clustering in time as well as space, and express a preference for the Jacquez test since it overcomes the need to specify critical space and time distances. Ward and Carpenter (2000) evaluate a number of space-time cluster tests to investigate possible clustering of blowfly catches on a commercial sheep property in Australia between 1997 and 1998. The tests compared include Jacquez's k nearest neighbour test (Jacquez 1996), the Knox test (Knox and Bartlett 1964), Mantel's test (Mantel 1967) and Barton's test (Barton et al. 1965). The Knox test indicates significant spatial (within 3 km) and temporal (within 1 month) clustering, which the other three tests do not identify. Ward and Carpenter (2000) use this to argue for the application of a number of different tests in cluster investigations. Jacquez's k nearest neighbour test can be implemented using the ClusterSeer software.

4.7 Conclusion

Clustering of a disease can occur for a variety of reasons, and the investigation of possible disease clustering is fundamental to epidemiology. The concepts and analytical methods discussed in this chapter take the epidemiologist beyond the mere visualization of spatial patterns as the use of statistical methods to assess whether observed patterns differ significantly from spatial randomness moves into the second stage of spatial analysis: that of exploration. Although the techniques outlined in this chapter are all estimates of global clustering, a sound understanding of their different methodologies, data requirements, and associated assumptions and limitations is essential if the most appropriate technique is to be chosen.

CHAPTER 5

Local estimates of spatial clustering

5.1 Introduction

Global measures of spatial association assume that the spatial process under investigation is stationary. Under this assumption, which is rarely met, global tests of association run the risk of obscuring local effects. As a result, significant local clustering may not be detected and conversely, large non-clustered areas within a study area may be ignored. The likelihood of including regions with inherently different local relationships increases as the size of the study area increases. With very large spatial datasets, and particularly with large raster datasets such as remotely sensed images, global statistics such as Moran's I (Moran 1948) run the risk of losing information on spatial autocorrelation since they summarize an enormous number of possibly dissimilar spatial relationships. Local statistics overcome this problem by scanning the entire dataset, but only measuring dependence in limited portions of the study area, the bounds of which have to be specified. Thus, for clustering to be detected, it need not occur over the entire dataset, nor need it have the same characteristics throughout the study area.

In studying local area clustering we are concerned with defining the characteristics of clusters, such as their location, size, and intensity. Knox (1989) proposes some definitions of clustering, one of which defines a cluster as 'a geographically and/or temporally bounded group of occurrences of sufficient size and concentration to be unlikely to have occurred by chance'. This purely statistical definition lends itself to this chapter. Whether these occurrences are due to some environmental, biological, or social variable (i.e. they are the direct

result of the distribution of risk factors) is the subject of Chapter 7.

The detection of disease clusters, particularly around putative point sources, has been the subject of much debate. In 1989 the Royal Statistical Society reported on a meeting held specifically to discuss the occurrence of cancer near nuclear installations (Muirhead and Darby 1989). The meeting was triggered by the highly popularized reports of excesses of childhood cancer, in particular leukaemia, around the reprocessing plants at Sellafield in Cumbria and Dounreay in northern Scotland. Its objective was to bring together epidemiologists (Doll 1989) and statisticians (Hills and Alexander 1989) to try and resolve whether excesses of cancer really were occurring in the vicinity of nuclear installations.

This triggered a spate of meetings, reported in Rothenberg et al. (1990), Lawson et al. (1995), Cliff (1995b), Jacquez et al. (1996), and Smith (1996). These addressed the legal aspects of disease cluster detection (Henderson 1990; Jacquez et al. 1992), and provided some useful reviews of statistical tests including those by Walter (1993), Waller and Turnbull (1993), Cliff (1995a), and Elliott et al. (1995).

In 1999 the Royal Statistical Society hosted an international conference on the 'analysis and interpretation of disease clusters and ecological studies' (Wakefield et al. 2001), during which the debate on whose method performs best was fuelled, old methodologies were adapted, and new methods introduced. Also addressed at this meeting were more philosophical questions such as when and how to investigate disease clusters, and indeed whether we should bother at all (Elliott and Wakefield 2001; Wartenberg 2001).

The complexity of the issues involving the public, media, local health authorities, epidemiologists, and those responsible for putative sources of increased incidence of disease, is exemplified in a case where the media reacted to documents released by the Ministry of Defence in 1977, disclosing simulation trials of germ warfare along the south coast of England between 1961 and 1977 (Stein 2001). Families in East Lulworth, a coastal village in Weymouth Bay, believed that exposure to the agents released during these trials had caused high rates of miscarriages, stillbirths, birth defects, and learning disabilities in the village. Under pressure from the media, campaigning families, environmental activists, and Members of Parliament the local health authority was forced to conduct a full scale investigation. No evidence of clustering could be found and the 'cluster that never was' was eventually refuted (Spratt 1999).

So 'cluster busting' has a long history and cuts into some difficult statistical, epidemiological, environmental, legal, and social territories. Cautious words on the interpretation of disease clustering studies are given by Besag and Newell (1991), Gardner (1992), Urquhart (1992), and Rothman (1990) who discuss some of the potential pitfalls surrounding cluster detection. Rothman (1990), for example, warns of the difficulties in defining the population base from which incidence rates can be calculated, and points out that due to high levels of publicity often surrounding such cases, unbiased data are difficult to collect. Rothman also warns that investigations into disease clusters are often made for political, rather than for scientific reasons and, quoting from Oakes (1986), that they are often based on significance tests that lack meaningful descriptive statistics and are prone to abuse and faulty inference. Urquhart (1992) highlights the risks of drawing conclusions about clustering (or its absence) in a particular area without knowledge of the underlying distribution of the disease. Besag and Newell (1991) point to the assumptions behind cluster detection tests, emphasizing that the null hypothesis must be based on equal and independent risk to each individual, and that the definition of the population at risk in terms of sex or age-group, and of geographical and temporal boundaries can have a profound impact on the outcome and significance levels. Gardner (1992) further emphasizes the risk of distorting estimates of disease excess, and of their significance levels, by *post hoc* selection of controls. He aptly describes the problem as 'moving the goalposts'.

Many texts have been written on the analysis of spatial point patterns. Examples include Cliff and Ord (1981), Upton and Fingleton (1985), Upton and Fingleton (1989), and Diggle (2003). Reviews of some of the available methods are provided by Marshall (1991a), Elliott et al. (1995), Morris and Wakefield (2000), Robinson (2000), Wakefield et al. (2000), Ward and Carpenter (2000), and Song and Kulldorff (2003). In this chapter some of the more commonly-used methods are reviewed. They are divided into those primarily designed for aggregated data, and those for point data, although this distinction is not rigid and most can be used with either type of data. Moreover, point data can easily be aggregated and area data can be represented as points, for example by using the centroids of the areas. The methods listed for point data are based on variously defined circles that 'scan' the data for areas of elevated (or reduced) disease frequency. Such statistics are better suited to point, than to area data, since points fall clearly inside or outside a scan circle. Scan circles can be defined in terms of geographic distance (e.g. Openshaw's method), number of cases (e.g. Besag and Newell's method) or population size (e.g. Turnbull's method and Kulldorff's scan statistic). Cluster detection is demonstrated by applying Kulldorff's scan statistic to the British cattle TB data. Methods for investigating clusters around point sources are then reviewed, and finally methods that look for clusters in both space and time. The space–time variant of Kulldorff's scan statistic is demonstrated using the British cattle TB data.

5.2 Methods for aggregated data

5.2.1 Getis and Ord's local Gi(d) statistic

Unlike Moran's I statistic (see Chapter 4), which measures the correlation between attribute values in adjacent areas, the Gi(d) local statistic (Getis and Ord 1992; 1996) is an indicator of local clustering that measures the 'concentration' of a spatially distributed attribute variable. Computational details of the of the $Gi(d)$ statistic are provided by Ding and Fotheringham (1992), Getis and Ord (1996), and Kitron et al. (1997). The test statistic is calculated as:

$$Gi(d) = \frac{\sum_{j}^{n} w_{ij}(d)(x_j - \bar{x}_i)}{S_i \sqrt{\frac{w_i(n-1-w_i)}{n-2}}}, \quad j \neq i \qquad (5.1)$$

where n is the number of areas within the region of interest and x_i is the observed value for area i

$$\bar{x}_i = \frac{1}{n-1} \sum_{j, \, j \neq i}^{n} x_j \qquad (5.2)$$

and w_{ij} is a symmetric binary spatial weights matrix:

$$w_i = \sum_{j, \, j \neq i}^{n} w_{ij} \qquad (5.3)$$

$$S_i^2 = \frac{1}{n-1} \sum_{j, \, j \neq i}^{n} (x_j - x_i)^2 \qquad (5.4)$$

It has been shown that $E(Gi) = 0$ and $\text{Var}(Gi) = 1$, and that the distribution of Gi under the null hypothesis of no spatial association among x_i is approximately normal (Ord and Getis 1993). By comparing local estimates of spatial autocorrelation with global averages, the $Gi(d)$ statistic identifies 'hotspots' in spatial data. The $Gi(d)$ statistic and a variety of other similar local statistics are discussed by Getis and Ord (1996), who also highlight some of their shortcomings, particularly those arising as a result of small sample sizes and the existence of high levels of global autocorrelation. Software to implement this statistic includes the spdep package in R, and ClusterSeer.

Getis and Ord (1992) use the $Gi(d)$ statistic to explore the spatial pattern of sudden infant death syndrome (SIDS) by county in North Carolina between 1979 and 1984. In addition to a number of small clusters, they identify a major hotspot in the mid-south of the state which they attribute to the distribution of health care facilities (Getis and Ord 1996). The general pattern of clustering is the same as that found by Grimson et al. (1981) using join count methods.

Kitron et al. (1997) use the $Gi(d)$ statistic to identify significant clustering of cases of La Crosse encephalitis over distances of 5 and 10 km, around particular towns in the Peoria area of Illinois. This analysis reveals a number of hotspots which they associate with homes on the edge of gullies and ravines where breeding and biting activities of the vector (*Aedes triseriatus*) are likely to occur.

Ding and Fotheringham (1992) developed the statistical analysis module (SAM) for ARC/INFO, based on the $Gi(d)$ local statistic. They use SAM to explore clustering of population growth in China between 1982 and 1990 and show that high rates of population growth are concentrated in the south. They attribute this to less severe restrictions on family size and greater proportions of ethnic minorities with large families in this region.

Moving towards exploring spatio-temporal clustering, Getis and Ord (1996) propose the use of local statistics to quantify the pattern and intensity of spread of a disease away from the core of a hotspot by estimating a series of local statistics at different time periods. Local statistics can be used to estimate the intensity of a disease at various distances from a core location, and the time dimension can then be used to estimate the rate of spread. Getis and Ord (1998) use the $Gi(d)$ statistic in this way to trace the spread of AIDS away from San Francisco.

5.2.2 Local Moran test

The local Moran test (Anselin 1995) detects local spatial autocorrelation in aggregated data by decomposing Moran's I statistic into contributions for each area within a study region. Termed Local Indicators of Spatial Association (LISA), the LISA statistic for each area is calculated as:

$$I_i = Z_i \sum_{j, \, j \neq i}^{n} w_{ij} Z_j \qquad (5.5)$$

where Z_i and Z_j are the observed values in standardized form, and w_{ij} is a spatial weights matrix in row-standardized form.

These indicators detect clusters of either similar or dissimilar disease frequency values around a given observation. The sum of the LISAs for all observations is proportional to the global Moran's I statistic. There are two uses of LISA statistics: either as indicators of local autocorrelation or as tests for outliers in global spatial patterns in the form of a Moran scatterplot (Anselin 1995; 1996). In a Moran scatterplot the horizontal axis represents the vector of observed values and the vertical axis specifies the weighted average of neighbouring values. The extent of the 'mix' of pairs among the four types of association in the quadrants of the plot defined by the axes (low–high, high–high, high–low and low–low) provides an indication of the stability of the spatial association throughout the data. It may also suggest the existence of different types of association in different subsets of the data; for example, positive association in one area and negative association in another. Software for implementing a local Moran test includes ClusterSeer, GeoDa, SpaceStat[40] and the spdep package in R.

Anselin (1995) demonstrates the local Moran test using patterns of conflict in Africa and compares it with Getis and Ord's local $Gi(d)$ statistic (Getis and Ord 1992). Anselin (1995) also developed LISAs for Mantel's test (Mantel 1967) and Geary's c (Geary 1954). The ClusterSeer and GeoDa software can be used to implement the LISA for Moran's I.

Burra et al. (2002) compare the ability of the local Moran test and Getis and Ord's local $Gi(d)$ statistic to detect clustering in mortality data from Hamilton, Ontario. These authors also evaluate the effect of geocoding errors on pattern detection, concluding that small geocoding errors can significantly influence the results of, and therefore the conclusions drawn from, these statistical tests. Jacquez and Greiling (2003) use the local Moran statistic to analyse spatial clustering in diagnoses of breast, lung, and colorectal cancers on Long Island, USA, identifying significant spatial patterns for all three diseases. Their analysis confirms the clustering of breast cancer mortality previously identified by Kulldorff et al. (1997) (see Section 5.3.4 for details of Kulldorff's spatial scan statistic), but they find that the two methods identify slightly different cluster locations. As a result of these differences Jacquez and Greiling (2003) recommend that a combination of statistics be used when studying local clustering

to ensure that different aspects of spatial patterns are identified and to check whether the results from different analyses are consistent. In a similar vein, Hanson and Wieczorek (2002) compare the local Moran statistic with Kulldorff's spatial scan statistic by exploring alcohol-related mortality in New York, USA. The clusters identified differ somewhat between the two methods and they conclude that the scan statistic is the more sensitive method. They advocate a multi-method approach to cluster detection since different methods tend to identify different characteristics of the clusters; the LISA identifying the core of a cluster and the scan statistic identifying its extent. A similar comparison is made by Nødtvedt et al. (2007) in an analysis of the spatial distribution of cases of atopic dermatitis in dogs in Sweden (1995–2000). They conclude that the tests produce similar results but that the LISA statistic identifies more localized clusters, compared to the larger clusters identified by the spatial scan statistic.

The following example continues on from the global Moran's I example presented in Section 4.4.1, which identified the existence of positive spatial autocorrelation among county-level TB-incidence rates in Britain in 1999 ($I = 0.0832$).

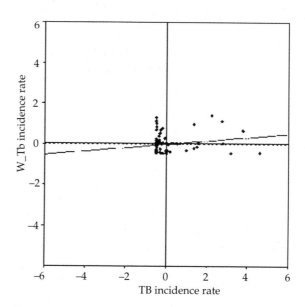

Figure 5.1 Moran scatterplot of county-level TB incidence rates in Britain in 1999.

Visual representation of this spatial autocorrelation can be obtained by applying the local Moran test to the data. Examination of the resulting Moran scatterplot (Fig 5.1) showed that most of the points were in the lower left (low-low) and upper left (low-high) quadrants indicating the existence of both positive and negative spatial autocorrelation among county level TB incidence rates in Britain in 1999; the negative spatial autocorrelation arising as a result of outlier counties with a low TB incidence rate being surrounded by neighbours with high TB incidence rates, while the positive spatial autocorrelation results from counties with a low TB incidence rate having neighbours with similar low incidence rates. The LISA cluster map and LISA significance map are additional, useful methods of visualising the spatial autocorrelation (and can be generated using the GeoDa software (Anselin et al. (2006)).

5.3 Methods for point data

5.3.1 Openshaw's Geographical Analysis Machine (GAM)

Openshaw's Geographical Analysis Machine (GAM) was the first in a series of methods developed to explore disease data for evidence of spatial pattern (Openshaw et al. 1987). The GAM involves applying a fine grid across a study area and generating a series of circles of varying radii with their centres based at each intersection of the grid. The observed number of cases of disease within each circle is then compared with the expected number of cases, assuming the process under investigation follows a Poisson distribution. Circles that have a higher than expected occurrence of disease are retained, resulting in a large number of overlapping circles concentrated around 'disease centres'. Visual inspection is then relied upon to decide where clusters occur. Further details and a quantitative treatment are provided in Openshaw et al. (1990). Openshaw's GAM can be implemented using the Dcluster package in R. Openshaw et al. (1988) and Turnbull et al. (1990) apply the GAM to investigate clustering of acute lymphoblastic leukaemia in northern England and leukaemia incidence in northern New York, respectively.

Statistical and computational limitations of the GAM methodology are described by Cuzick and Edwards (1990), Turnbull et al. (1990), Marshall (1991a), and Besag and Newell (1991). The main criticism of the technique is that it does not account for multiple testing, and therefore the change in radius and shifts in location of candidate clusters are not taken into account in the calculation of significance levels. Despite having being widely criticized, the GAM seems to have inspired the development of a series of tests for cluster detection based on scan circles, which have addressed and overcome many of the deficiencies of the original GAM, gradually adapting and improving upon its basic methodology.

5.3.2 Turnbull's Cluster Evaluation Permutation Procedure (CEPP)

Turnbull et al. (1990) developed the first test that was able to both locate and test the significance of disease clusters. The test, called the Cluster Evaluation Permutation Procedure (CEPP), creates a circular window for each area that contains a pre-determined number of individuals at risk, R. The number of individuals at risk in an area can be defined as p_i and the number of disease events as O_i. If the number of individuals at risk (p_i), is less than R, then area i is included in the window and the area whose centroid is nearest to that of area i (say cell j) is included if $O_i + O_j < R$. If $O_i + O_j > R$ a fraction of the population of area j is added so that the total population at risk equals R. If $O_i > R$ then the window contains only a fraction of area i. For the fractional area included in a window, cases are allocated in the same proportion to the window as that of the population of the cell. A series of i overlapping windows is created with a population at risk of constant size, R. Turnbull's test statistic, as a function of R, equals the maximum number of cases in each of the windows. Monte Carlo simulation is used to evaluate the significance of the observed test statistic. Software for implementing the CEPP includes the Dcluster package in R, and ClusterSeer.

One of the conditions of this procedure is that cluster size (in terms of number of individuals at risk) must be defined *a priori* for the procedure to be valid. Turnbull et al. (1990) apply the CEPP to leukaemia incidence data obtained from the New York State Cancer Registry, for an upstate New York region comprising eight contiguous counties, and compare its performance with Openshaw's GAM, concluding that the main advantage of the CEPP over the GAM is that it provides a quantitative assessment of the statistical significance of identified clusters.

5.3.3 Besag and Newell's method

One disadvantage of the GAM is that, since distance is the method used to define the scan circles, circles of the same size can refer to different-sized populations and are therefore not directly comparable. Besag and Newell (1991) developed a method to rectify this problem whereby the user specifies k, the expected cluster size. Typical values for k range between 2 and 10 for rare diseases. Each area with non-zero cases is considered in turn as the centre of a possible cluster. When evaluating an area it is labelled as 0 and the remaining areas are ordered according to their distance from area 0 and labelled 1, 2,..., $i - 1$. Using the notation defined in the previous section (O_i is the number of disease events) the statistic D_i is calculated such that $D_i = \sum_{j=0}^{i} O_j$ O_j and $D_0 \leq D_1 \leq \dots$ are the accumulated number of cases in cells 0, 1, ... and $u_0 \leq u_1 \leq \dots$ are the corresponding accumulated number of individuals at risk. $M = \min \{i: D_i \geq k\}$ so that the nearest M areas contain the closest k cases. A small observed value of M indicates a cluster centred at cell 0. If m is the observed value of M, then the significance level of each potential cluster is:

$$\Pr\{M \leq m\} = 1 - \sum_{s=0}^{k-1} \exp(-u_m Q) \qquad (5.6)$$
$$(u_m Q)^s / s!$$

where Q equals the total number of cases in the study area divided by the total population at risk. The test statistic of clustering in the study area, T_{BN}, equals the total number of individually significant clusters, for example, at p < 0.05. The significance of the observed T_{BN} can be determined by Monte Carlo simulation. Further details of the methodology are provided by Besag and Newell (1991) and Alexander and Cuzick (1992). Software for implementing Besag and Newell's test includes the Dcluster package in R, and ClusterSeer.

Two limitations of this method, common to many other cluster detection tests are firstly, the *a priori* choice of cluster size and secondly, the problem of multiple testing arising from the large number of potential clusters. Since the calculations to determine significance are based on the specified number of nearest-neighbour cases, selecting its value is an important issue. If it is too small then larger clusters cannot be detected, and if it is too large spurious clusters may be identified (Le et al. 1996). Besag and Newell (1991) demonstrate their methodology using data for acute lymphoblastic leukaemias in children under the age of 14 years in part of the Mersey Regional Health Authority Districts of England (1975–1985). They identify 23 clusters significant at the 5% level, which fall into seven discrete groups. Interestingly, and in agreement with the Black Report (Black 1984), they find no evidence of clustering in the vicinity of the Sellafield nuclear reprocessing plant during this period (see Section 5.4 for more details on this issue).

Alexander et al. (1991) adapted Besag and Newell's method into the nearest neighbour areas (NNA) test for local clustering (formulae are provided in Alexander et al. (1991)). They apply the NNA test to data on the incidence of selected childhood cancers and to adult haematopoietic malignancies in Yorkshire, UK, confirming an unusual distribution of lymphoma in Yorkshire associated with the North Yorkshire moors. Alexander et al. (1989) apply the NNA test to data on the incidence of Hodgkin's disease in England and Wales (1984–1986), finding weak but significant evidence of localized spatial clustering, particularly in young adults.

Fotheringham and Zhan (1996) review and compare the tests developed by Openshaw and Besag and Newell. These authors use a database on housing quality in the city of Amherst, New York, containing 277 very low quality residences among the total population of 28,832. By using the two different methods to identify clusters of low quality residences they conclude that, although both tests perform reasonably well in identifying genuine clusters, the specificity of Besag and Newell's test is superior to that of the GAM.

More recently Huillard d'Aignaux et al. (2002) use Besag and Newell's method to explore the possibility of spatial clustering in sporadic Creutzfeldt-Jakob disease (CJD) in France between 1992 and 1998, identifying five clusters that were persistent over a range of values of k. Only one of these clusters is identified by Kulldorff's scan statistic (see Section 5.3.4). Using a simulated benchmark dataset Marcelo and Renato (2005) compare Besag and Newell's test with Kulldorff's scan statistic, finding that they give similar results but that the scan statistic is more likely to identify clusters in sparsely populated areas.

5.3.4 Kulldorff's spatial scan statistic

Inspired by Openshaw's GAM (Openshaw et al. 1987) and a generalization of Turnbull's CEPP (Turnbull et al. 1990), Kulldorff developed the spatial scan statistic (Kulldorff and Nagarwalla 1995), which brings together the advantages of each technique. For each specified location a series of circles of varying radii is constructed. Each circle absorbs the nearest neighbouring locations that fall inside it and the radius of each circle is set to increase continuously from zero until some fixed percentage of the total population is included. For each circle the alternative hypothesis is that there is an elevated risk of disease within the circle compared to that outside (Kulldorff et al. 1998b). The test statistic T_{KN} is calculated as:

$$T_{KN} = \sup_Z \left(\frac{O(Z)}{p(Z)} \right)^{n(Z)} \left(\frac{O(Z^c)}{p(Z^c)} \right)^{n(Z^c)}$$
$$I\left(\frac{O(Z)}{p(Z)} > \frac{O(Z^c)}{p(Z^c)} \right) \tag{5.7}$$

where Z^c indicates all circles except for Z, $O()$ and $p()$ are the observed number of cases and the population size in each area respectively, and $I(.)$ is the indicator function. Monte Carlo simulation is conducted to compare T_{KN}, with the distribution of values generated under the null hypothesis.

Kulldorff (1997) implemented the spatial scan statistic in a cluster detection programme called

SaTScan[41], which searches for clusters in datasets using two different probabilistic models; a Bernoulli model where cases and controls are compared as Boolean variables, and a Poisson model where the number of cases is compared to the background population data and the expected number of cases in each unit is proportional to the size of the population at risk. Circle centres are defined either by the case and control/population data or by specifying an array of grid coordinates. Secondary clusters are computed, based on the degree of overlap allowed in the cluster circles, and includes the options no geographical overlap, and no cluster centres in other clusters. Software for implementing the spatial scan statistic includes SaTScan, the Dcluster package in R, and ClusterSeer.

Until recently a major limitation of the spatial scan statistic was the use of a circular scanning window which decreased the likelihood of the statistic detecting non-circular clusters. However, the most recent version of SaTScan can implement an elliptic version of the spatial scan statistic, which uses a scanning window of variable location, shape, angle and size, thereby greatly increasing the ability of the statistic to detect non-circular clusters (Kulldorff et al. 2006b). Choosing the shape of the ellipsoid will depend on the nature of the data and the questions being asked, and the authors stress that the type of ellipsoid to be used must be chosen before looking at the data in order to prevent any pre-selection bias. For example, a long, narrow ellipsoid might be used to investigate potential clusters along a riverbank. The circular and elliptic scan statistics have similar power, with the circular scan statistic able to detect elliptic clusters and *vice versa*, although the elliptic scan statistic may provide a better estimate of the true area of the cluster. Although the elliptic scan statistic is more flexible than the circular scan statistic it still imposes a shape on potential clusters and therefore, for irregularly-shaped clusters (e.g. along a winding river) it may be more appropriate to use one of the non-parametric spatial scan statistics described in Section 5.3.5.

Kulldorff and Nagarwalla (1995) use the spatial scan statistic, based on a Bernoulli model, to detect clusters of leukaemia cases in northern New York,

---

[41] http://www.satscan.org

USA. The results of this analysis are compared with a number of other cluster-detection algorithms, including those of Turnbull et al. (1990) and Openshaw et al. (1987). One primary cluster and four non-overlapping secondary clusters are identified in similar locations to those identified visually using Openshaw's GAM in an analysis of the same data (Turnbull et al. 1990).

Hanson and Wieczorek (2002) use the spatial scan statistic (which they compare to a LISA, see Section 5.2.2) in a study of alcohol-related mortality in New York, USA. Huillard d'Aignaux et al. (2002) explore the possibility of spatial clustering of sporadic CJD in France between 1992 and 1998. Using the spatial scan statistic they identify only one significant cluster of sporadic CJD yet identify five disease clusters using Besag and Newell's method. Kulldorff et al. (2003) find the spatial scan statistic performs well when compared against two global tests, Tango's maximized excess events test (Tango 1995; 2000) and the nonparametric M statistic (Bonetti and Pagano 2004), on a collection of simulated datasets generated under different cluster models. They encourage other investigators to contribute to a common bank of cluster-simulation datasets, and to use this collection as a benchmark against which to evaluate both existing and new cluster-detection tests.

Early applications of the scan statistic include an investigation of childhood leukaemia in Sweden (Hjalmars et al. 1996) in which no evidence was found to support previous assertions of disease clustering. Kulldorff et al. (1997) demonstrate clustering of breast cancer mortality in the northeastern part of the USA (1988–1992) after adjusting for confounding variables such as age, race, urbanicity, and parity.

Recuenco et al. (2007) compare clustering of enzootic racoon rabies in New York State (1997–2003) under different regimes of covariate adjustment: (i) no adjustment, (ii) adjustment for landscape covariates, and (iii) adjustment for landscape covariates and large-scale geographic variation. Clusters identified under the unadjusted test regime tend to also be identified in the covariate-adjusted analyses, though some drop from significance. They use these differences in clusters identified under the three regimes to make inferences regarding the possible reasons for high-risk areas.

The spatial scan statistic has now been applied to an impressive range of health-related problems[42]. This is due in part to its addressing many of the problems of earlier scan statistics but also because SaTScan, the freely available primary software for implementing the spatial scan statistic, makes it accessible to a wide, non-specialized audience. There is insufficient space here to review these works in detail (although salient points are raised where appropriate) but the method has been applied to identify clustering in a variety of cancers (Viel et al. 2000; Jemal et al. 2002; Roche et al. 2002; Boscoe et al. 2003; Buntinx et al. 2003; Gregorio and Samociuk 2003; Klassen et al. 2005; Jung et al. 2006), sexually transmitted diseases (Jennings et al. 2005; Wylie et al. 2005); variant CJD (Cousens et al. 2001), systemic lupus erythematosus (SLE) (Walsh and DeChello 2001), human granulocytic ehrlichiosis (HGE) (Chaput et al. 2002), insulin-dependent diabetes mellitus (Green et al. 2003), childhood mortality (Sankoh et al. 2001), low birth rate (Ozdenerol et al. 2005), congenital malformations (Forand et al. 2002), SIDS (George et al. 2001), highland malaria (Brooker et al. 2004), and systemic sclerosis (Walsh and Fenster 1997). In the veterinary literature the method has been applied to psoroptic sheep scab (Falconi et al. 2002), bovine TB (Perez et al. 2002; Olea-Popelka et al. 2003; Olea-Popelka et al. 2005), BSE (Stevenson et al. 2000; Abrial et al. 2003), sylvatic plague agents in coyotes (Hoar et al. 2003), toxoplasma infections in sea otters (Miller et al. 2002; 2004a), and atopic dermatitis in dogs (Nødtvedt et al. 2007), to name but a few.

5.3.5 Non-parametric spatial scan statistics

A significant restriction imposed by all of the methods reviewed here is that they assume disease clusters are circular. As these conditions seldom occur in reality, attempts have recently been made to overcome this problem by developing a variety of tests that can locate irregularly-shaped disease clusters, including those described by Duczmal and Assunção (2004), Patil and Taillie (2004), Tango and Takahashi (2005), and Duczmal et al. (2006).

Spatial scan statistics use circles for the scanning window, that have a low power for detecting

[42] http://www.satscan.org/references.html

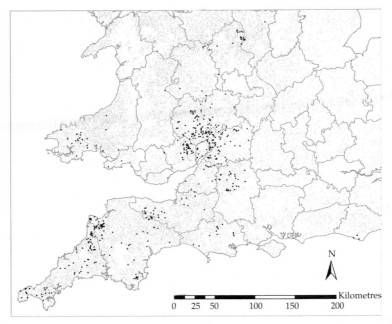

Figure 5.2 Distribution of herds (small grey spots) and tuberculosis breakdowns (large black spots) in the southwest of Britain in 1997.

irregularly-shaped clusters, and may in fact identify an irregularly-shaped cluster as a series of small circular clusters. In an attempt to overcome this and other limitations of spatial scan statistics Patil and Taillie (2004) developed the upper level set scan statistic which they apply to three ecological situations in order to illustrate its uses: the early detection of biological invasions, mapping vegetative disturbance, and the characterization of biological impairment of rivers and streams in Pennsylvania.

Duczmal and Assunção (2004) use a simulated annealing approach to identify 'connected clusters with arbitrary shape'. However, Tango and Takahashi (2005) suggest that although Duczmal and Assunção's (2004) test can detect irregularly-shaped clusters, they are much larger than the true clusters and they therefore developed a flexibly shaped spatial scan statistic for detecting irregular-shaped clusters within small areas of a region. This statistic works well at detecting small circular and non-circular clusters (Tango and Takahashi, 2005) and can be implemented using the FlexScan software.[43]

[43] http://www.niph.go.jp/soshiki/gijutsu/download/flexscan/index.html

5.3.6 Example of local cluster detection

To demonstrate local cluster detection Kulldorff's spatial scan statistic was applied to the British cattle TB breakdown herd data (1986–1997). Due to the nature of the TB data (see Chapter 1), incidence rates cannot be accurately derived, and therefore the analysis was restricted to the use of the Bernoulli model. All TB breakdown herds were included as cases, and compared against a sample of control herds (due to computer memory limitations) and the combined data were used to define the circle centres for cluster detection (rather than specifying a special set of grid coordinates). Based on some preliminary analyses a 30% sample of control herds was chosen, above which no real change in the pattern of clustering occurred. The most restrictive option was selected for dealing with overlapping clusters, in which secondary clusters were reported only if they did not overlap with a previously reported cluster.

Fig. 5.2 shows the distribution of herds (small grey dots) and of breakdown herds (larger black dots) in the southwest of Britain in 1997. In order to compare various options for implementing the spatial scan statistic, the 1997 dataset was used as this was the year with most recorded breakdowns (amongst those years within the dataset).

The single most important subjective choice that has to be made when using the spatial scan statistic is specification of the maximum percentage of the population at risk (between 1 and 50%) that can be included in any one cluster. The SaTScan manual (Kulldorff 2003) recommends specifying a high upper limit (i.e. 50%) of the population at risk, since SaTScan will then look for clusters of both small and large sizes without any pre-selection bias in terms of the cluster size. When looking for clusters of high rates a cluster of larger size indicates areas of exceptionally low rates outside the circle rather than an area of exceptionally high rates within the circle. A review of the literature reveals that most authors do not indicate the upper limit specified in their analyses, presumably using the default value of 50%. Studies stating explicitly that an upper limit of 50% was selected include Walsh and Fenster (1997), George et al. (2001), Huillard d'Aignaux et al. (2002), Roche et al. (2002), Brooker et al. (2004), and Schwermer et al. (2007). A variety of values below this are also reported including 10% by Norström et al. (2000) (to avoid scanning outside the geographic region of the study), 10% by Sheehan et al. (2000) (no reason given), 3.4% by Walsh and DeChello (2001) (based on the population size of the largest county in their study), 5% by Falconi et al. (2002) (no reason given), 2.5% by Forand et al. (2002) (in order to provide better focus on geographical areas for further evaluation and follow up), 5% by Sauders et al. (2003) (no reason given), and 25% by Recuenco et al. (2007) (no reason given).

The results of specifying different upper limits for cluster size when using the British cattle TB data for 1997 (with a 30% sample of control herds) are shown in Fig. 5.3 in which the selected upper limits were (a) 1%, (b) 5%, (c) 10%, (d) 20%, (e) 30% and (f) 50%.

The 1% upper limit produced ten highly significant (p < 0.001) and ten less significant (1.0 > p > 0.001) clusters. The 50% upper limit produced one enormous, highly significant cluster, one tiny highly significant cluster and one very small, less significant cluster. Moving from an upper limit of 1% towards one of 50% produced smaller numbers of increasingly large and increasingly significant clusters. Which of these patterns of clustering best

reflects the epidemiology of TB in the southwest of Britain cannot be determined from this analysis.

To explore the outcomes of the cluster analysis in greater detail consider Table 5.1 and the associated Fig. 5.4. Table 5.1 shows some statistics for the (arbitrarily chosen) 5% maximum cluster size of the 1997 TB data (Fig. 5.3b).

It is quite clear that, as suggested by Boscoe et al. (2003), some of the most significant clusters are of relatively low risk and *vice versa*. Cluster 8 for example, has by far the highest prevalence but is barely significant, while the similarly sized Cluster 3 also has a high prevalence but is highly significant. The very large, highly significant and so called primary cluster (Cluster 1), only has a relatively low prevalence.

Fig. 5.4 illustrates these points through two contrasting representations of the analysis: the log likelihood ratio, which indicates the probability of a cluster being real (Fig. 5.4a), and the prevalence (Fig. 5.4b), which is directly proportional to the relative risk within a cluster but corrected for sampling of the population.

Cluster analysis was conducted for each year from 1986 to 1997. Non-overlapping clusters were identified using the Bernoulli model with all TB breakdown herds as cases compared against 30% of control herds and a maximum cluster size set to 5% of all points. Fig. 5.5 shows the evolution of TB clusters during this period. Annual clustering of TB breakdowns is represented by the log likelihood ratios, using the same scale for each year. For most of the period two large and highly significant clusters were fairly constant. These were Cluster 1 (as labelled in Fig. 5.4) on the Gloucestershire, Hereford, and Worcester boundaries, and Cluster 2 on the Devon/Cornwall boundary. Cluster 7 in Dyfed in western Wales is much smaller and of lower significance but is persistent, falling from significance only during 1987 and 1989. Some clusters tended to appear, disappear, and then re-appear in much the same place. For example, Cluster 8 in East Sussex was apparent between 1989 and 1991, in 1994 and again in 1997, while Cluster 3 on the Staffordshire/Derbyshire boundary was first evident briefly in 1993 and then re-emerged between 1996 and 1997. Perhaps these are the main centres of endemicity that act as sources of infection via, for

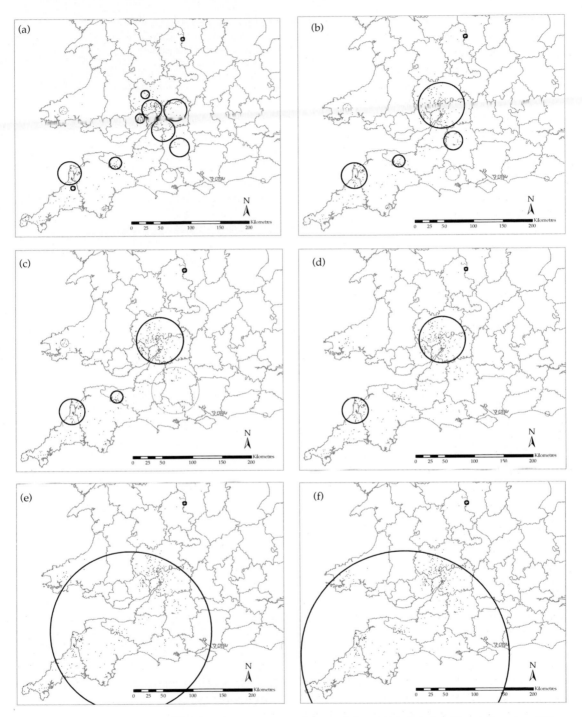

Figure 5.3 Cluster analysis comparing different maximum percentages of the population at risk to be included in a cluster, using all TB breakdown herds as cases and a 30% sample of control herds, in the southwest of Britain, in 1977. Maximum percentage of the population at risk to be included in clusters was a) 1%, b) 5%, c) 10%, d) 20%, e) 30% and f) 50%. Bold black circles indicate P-values of < 0.001; fine grey circles indicate P-values between 0.001 and 1.00.

Table 5.1 Details of the spatial clusters illustrated in Figures 5.3.b and 5.4. For each cluster the area is given, LLR is the log likelihood ratio, P (999) is the significance level based on 999 Monte Carlo replications (hence the plateau at 0.001), RR is the relative risk (observed/expected), which is directly proportional to Prev., (the prevalence corrected for sampling)

Cluster	Area (km²)	LLR	P (999)	RR	Prev.
1	4,879	280.5	0.001	8.3	0.048
2	1,516	115.8	0.001	9.7	0.056
3	32	33.7	0.001	35.7	0.206
4	821	32.6	0.001	7.3	0.042
5	337	32.4	0.001	11.2	0.065
6	37	18.4	0.002	20.8	0.120
7	149	14.4	0.010	8.2	0.048
8	52	13.3	0.030	41.6	0.240
9	479	12.5	0.052	7.8	0.048
10	82	9.7	0.427	15.3	0.088

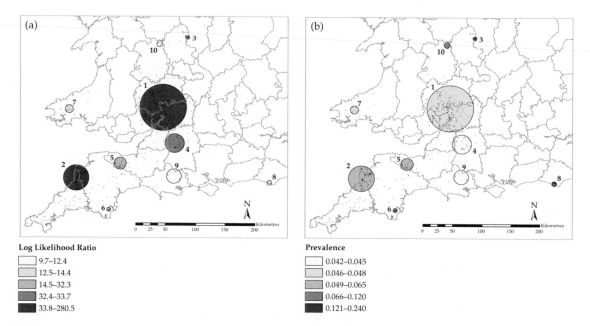

Log Likelihood Ratio
- 9.7–12.4
- 12.5–14.4
- 14.5–32.3
- 32.4–33.7
- 33.8–280.5

Prevalence
- 0.042–0.045
- 0.046–0.048
- 0.049–0.065
- 0.066–0.120
- 0.121–0.240

Figure 5.4 Detailed cluser analysis showing a) log likelihood ratios (i.e. probability) and b) prevalence (directly proportional to relative risk) of clusters of TB breakdown herds in the southwest of Britain, in 1977. Clusters were identified using the Bernoulli model using all TB breakdown herds as cases compared to 30% of control heads, with a maximum cluster size set to 5% of all points. See also Figure 5.3.b and Table 5.1.

example, cattle movements (Gilbert et al. 2005) into areas where prevailing environmental and epidemiological conditions allow new disease clusters to arise, as indicated for example in Wint et al. (2002). Clearly there are clusters of bovine TB in the southwest of Britain, some persistent, some fleeting, and some recurring.

5.4 Detecting clusters around a source (focused tests)

With focused tests the location of a cluster centre is specified *a priori*, and the likelihood of that location truly being a cluster centre is then determined. Localized clustering of disease around

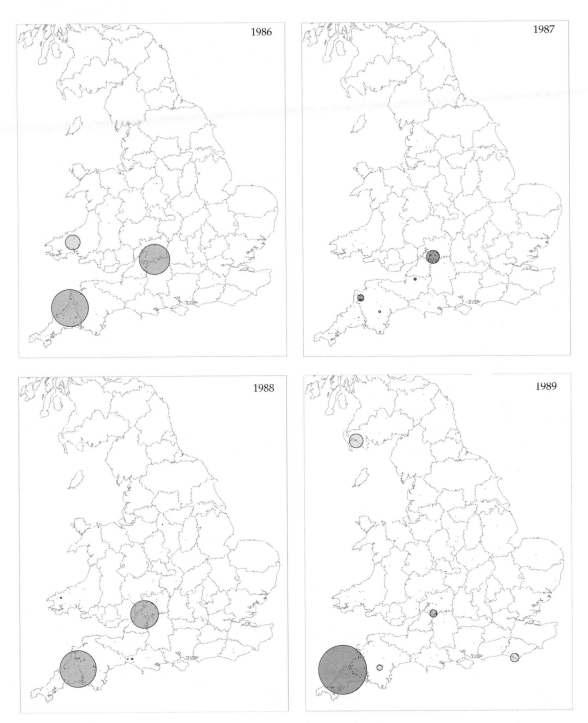

Figure 5.5 Cluster analysis of cattle TB data (1986–1997). Clusters were identified for each year using the spatial scan statistic and the Bernoulli model with all TB breakdown herds compared to 30% of control herds, with a maximum cluster size set to 5% of all points and no overlapping clusters permitted. Clusters are shaded by log likelihood ratio using the same scale for each year with darker clusters being the most likely. The distribution of breakdown herds in each year is superimposed on the cluster map.

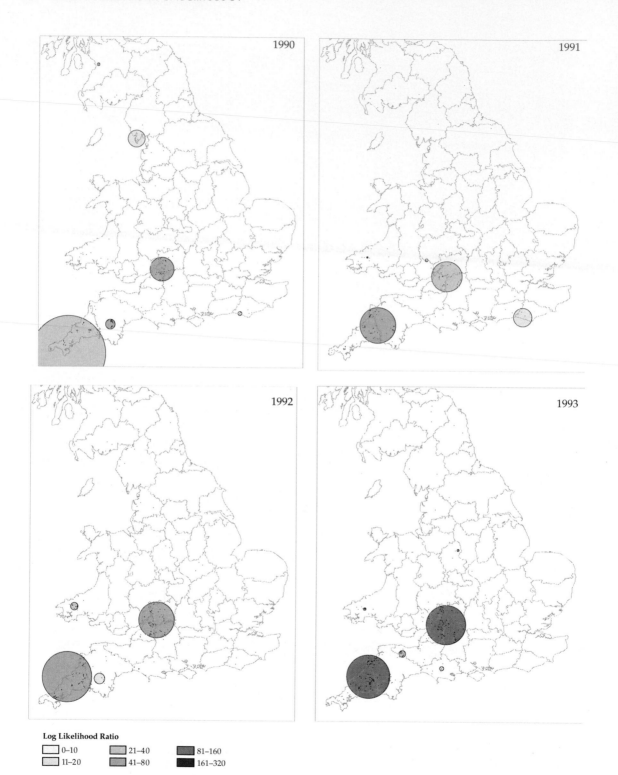

Log Likelihood Ratio

☐ 0–10	☐ 21–40	◼ 81–160
☐ 11–20	☐ 41–80	◼ 161–320

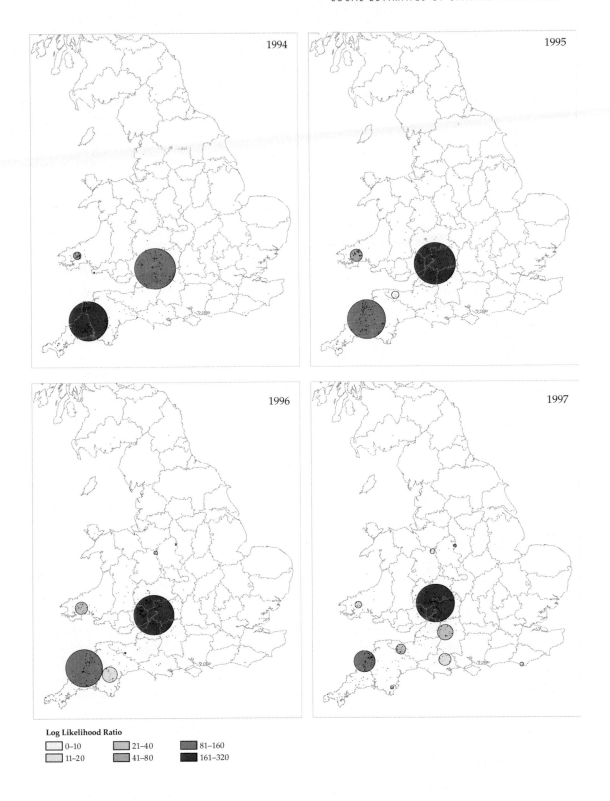

Log Likelihood Ratio

- 0–10
- 11–20
- 21–40
- 41–80
- 81–160
- 161–320

environmental hazards is a sensitive issue, exemplified by the highly publicized investigations into elevated childhood leukaemia incidence around the Sellafield nuclear reprocessing plant in the 1980s. Suspicions were aroused by researchers for a television company in 1983 (Gardner 1989; 1992). The Yorkshire Television programme 'Windscale, the nuclear laundry', alleged that elevated levels of childhood leukaemia resulted from nuclear discharge from the plant into the Irish Sea, leading to a Government inquiry that resulted in the Black Report (Black 1984). This report confirmed a high incidence of cancer in the study area, which it maintained is 'unusual but not unique', and that no causal link between nuclear power and illness could be proved. Not surprisingly this sparked debate into the validity of the statistical methods applied and initiated a series of investigations into cancer clusters around nuclear and other 'high risk' sites (reviewed by Alexander and Boyle (2000)). Caldwell (1990) reports that investigations into 108 space–time clusters during 22 years of cancer cluster investigations at the Centres for Disease Control and Prevention in the United States, showed no consistent patterns or clues as to disease aetiology, and Alexander and Boyle (2000) state that 'whilst many statistically significant clusters have been identified, none has ever been explained by an environmental pollutant or infectious agent'.

Comprehensive reviews on cluster detection around putative point sources have been written, including those by Hills and Alexander (1989), Muirhead and Darby (1989), Marshall (1991a), Elliott et al. (1995), and Morris and Wakefield (2000). It is not the intention to go into great detail here, but rather to provide an overview. Morris and Wakefield (2000) provide a useful review of a variety of methods, applying them to a single example; the incidence of stomach cancer in relation to proximity to a municipal solid-waste incinerator in Great Britain (see also Elliott et al. (1996)). Besag and Newell (1991) warn against pre-selection bias arising from a point source being chosen for investigation based on a prior knowledge of a higher disease incidence in its vicinity. Hills and Alexander (1989) distinguish between situations where there is a prior hypothesis about a source and those where the hypothesis is reactive. They emphasize the

problem of choosing the area around the source, and of accommodating extra-Poisson variability. Wartenberg and Greenberg (1993) highlight the importance of choosing appropriate techniques for given circumstances. In specifying the null hypothesis, usually that the disease events occur with a uniformly distributed probability of risk, they emphasize the importance of choosing a method that can account for any confounding variables such as age, gender, occupation, or ethnicity. In determining the alternative hypothesis they stress the importance of different clinical patterns of disease resulting from a single risk source as opposed to more general hotspots.

5.4.1 Stone's test

Stone (1988) developed a class of tests for trend, the maximum likelihood ratio (MLR) and Poisson maximum (Pmax) tests, both of which use the first isotonic regression estimator, working on the assumption that there will be a monotonic decay of risk with increasing distance from any point-source of a disease. Stone's Pmax test is applied to data on cancer incidence in the vicinities of the Siezewell and Sellafield nuclear installations (Bithell and Stone 1989). At Sellafield they demonstrate a highly significant trend in disease excess indicating a genuine association, but geographical proximity to the power station at Seascale does not appear to be important. Software for implementing Stone's test includes the Dcluster package in R.

Elliott et al. (1992b) use Stone's test to analyse the incidence of lung and laryngeal cancer around incinerators of waste solvents and oils at Charnock Richard in Lancashire (1972–1980), but find no evidence for a decreasing risk of cancer with increasing distance from the sites. In a later study Elliott et al. (1996) examine an extended cancer dataset for Great Britain in relation to solid-waste incinerators, finding no evidence for declining risk with distance from incinerators for cancer of the larynx or connective tissues (including soft-tissue sarcoma), nasal and nasopharyngeal cancer, and non-Hodgkin lymphomas. However, significant results are obtained for all cancers combined, and for stomach, colorectal, liver, and lung cancers, although these results are thought to be due to confounding effects such as deprivation.

Stone's test has been applied to studies of cancer incidence near radio and television transmitters. In a study specific to the Sutton Coldfield transmitter in Great Britain, Dolk et al. (1997b) find the risk of adult leukaemia between 1974 and 1986 to be elevated within 2 km of the transmitter, and to decline significantly with increasing distance from the transmitter. They extend this study to explore the incidence of cancers in the vicinity of 20 high-power transmitters across Great Britain (1974–1986) (Dolk et al. 1997a) and whilst they do find evidence for a declining leukaemia risk with increasing distance from transmitters, conclude that the pattern around the Sutton Coldfield transmitter is uncommon. Michelozzi et al. (2002) use Stone's test to investigate the incidence of adult and childhood leukaemia in the vicinity of the Vatican Radio high-power radio transmitter. The result is significant for children and male adults, with a declining risk as a function of distance from the transmitter, but no explanation is provided for these findings.

A number of adaptations of the original method have been developed. For example, Morton-Jones et al. (1999) propose an extension that allows for covariate adjustments via a log-linear model, which they illustrate using data on the incidence of stomach cancers near municipal incinerators. Diggle et al. (1999) adapted Stone's isotonic regression method to incorporate case-control data in addition to covariate information. They illustrate the adaptations using data on lung and laryngeal cancers in the vicinity of an industrial incinerator, and on childhood asthma in relation to distance from major roads. Consistent with Diggle (1990) they show moderate evidence of increased risk of cancer of the larynx in the vicinity of the disused industrial incinerator, compared with the more common incidence of lung cancer, in the Chorley-Ribble area of south Lancashire, England between 1974 and 1983, although covariate information is not available for this dataset. They also find no association between asthma in children in North Derbyshire in 1992 and distance from major roads, after adjusting for the covariates of age and sex (in agreement with Diggle and Rowlingson (1994)).

5.4.2 The Lawson–Waller score test

Lawson (1993) and Waller et al. (1992) developed the Lawson–Waller score test, sometimes referred to as the uniformly most powerful (UMP) test. The score test detects a decreasing trend in disease frequency associated with declining exposure to a point-focus. The test statistic T_{LW} is given by:

$$T_{LW} = \sum_{i=1}^{I} g_i(O_i - E_i) \tag{5.8}$$

$$Var(T_{LW}) = \sum_{i=1}^{I} g_i^2 E_i - O_i \left(\sum_{i=1}^{I} \frac{p_i g_i}{p_+} \right)^2 \tag{5.9}$$

where g_i denotes the exposure to the focus for an individual residing in area i, O_i is the observed number of disease cases in area i, E_i is the expected number of disease cases in area i, p_i is the size of the population at risk in area i, and p_+ is the total population size. Monte Carlo simulation is used to evaluate the significance of the test statistic T_{LW}.

Waller et al. (1992) demonstrate the methodology using leukaemia incidence data in upstate New York (1978–1982), with waste sites containing trichloroethylene as putative hazardous point-sources. Lawson (1993) demonstrates the methodology using bronchitis mortality around a chemical reprocessing plant in Bonnybridge, central Scotland (1980–1982).

Michelozzi et al. (2002) apply the Lawson–Waller score test to investigate the incidence of adult and childhood leukaemia in the vicinity of the Vatican Radio high-power radio transmitter. Waller et al. (1992), Waller and Turnbull (1993), Waller and Lawson (1995), and Waller (1996) compare the Lawson–Waller score test with Besag and Newell's test (Besag and Newell 1991) (adapted as a focused clustering test) and with Stone's test (Stone 1988), concluding that the sensitivity of the methods depends on the level of aggregation of the underlying surveillance data (Waller 1996). From a number of simulations to compare the power of each test they conclude that for very rare diseases all tests have low power, with Stone's test performing least well, followed by Besag and Newell's test, and that the best by a small margin was the Lawson–Waller score test. Increasing the disease prevalence improved the power of all the tests. In this instance the power of Stone's test surpasses that of Besag and Newell's test. They conclude that their own test outperforms the other two, in terms of power, under all conditions.

5.4.3 Bithell's linear risk score tests

Bithell et al. (1994) and Bithell (1995) developed a set of tests known as 'linear risk score tests', where disease incidence is weighted by some distance function from a point source (e.g. $1/d_i$, $1/d_i^2$, or $1/rank_i$). Using the reciprocal of distance is appropriate for detecting an environmental hazard that declines with distance from a source and is relatively insensitive to the precise location of the assumed source. Using the reciprocal of rank is more appropriate when the relative proximity of residence is important, rather than actual distance, but it is more sensitive to the precise location of the putative source. Bithell et al. (1994) compare the power of these tests against Stone's Pmax and MLR tests concluding that they are likely to be more powerful than Stone's tests, particularly in situations where non-uniformity of risk is only slight. They apply these tests to the distribution of childhood leukaemia around 23 nuclear installations in England and Wales (Bithell 1995) with only two, Sellafield and Burghfield, giving significant results. They conclude that there is no evidence for a general increase in childhood leukaemia in the vicinity of nuclear installations, and that apart from Sellafield, the evidence for distance-related risk is weak. Bithell's linear risk score tests can be implemented using the ClusterSeer software.

5.4.4 Diggle's test

Diggle (1990) developed a test that uses nonparametric kernel smoothing to describe natural variation in a disease (assuming a Poisson point process), and then a maximum likelihood test to evaluate the possibility of raised incidence around a pre-specified point source. Diggle (1990) demonstrates the approach, exploring links between a disused industrial incinerator and a possibly elevated incidence of laryngeal cancers, compared with the more common incidence of lung cancer, in the Chorley-Ribble area of south Lancashire. Kernel smoothing is used to describe the more common lung cancer

incidence, providing an estimate of 'natural' spatial variation. A parametric maximum likelihood approach is then used to describe raised incidence in laryngeal cancer near the pre-specified source. This clustering is confirmed using Monte Carlo simulations. Diggle and Rowlingson (1994) developed a conditional approach, which converts the original point process model into a non-linear binary regression model for the spatial variation in risk. Using the same cancer datasets from south Lancashire they show similar results but conclude that these should be more reliable than those obtained from the original point process model. Moreover, this adaptation allows adjustment for covariates in a log-linear fashion. They further demonstrate the method using asthma data from North Derbyshire in 1992. Three putative point sources; a coking works, a chemical plant, and a waste treatment centre, are evaluated after adjusting for a number of covariates including distance from roads, presence of a cigarette-smoker in the household, dust problems, and hay fever. They find some evidence for association with the coking works and a significant association with the presence of hay fever. Software for implementing Diggle's test includes the splancs package in R, and ClusterSeer.

5.4.5 Kulldorff's focused spatial scan statistic

The spatial scan statistic can be used to search for clusters around a point source by making the point source the only coordinate pair in the special grid file. In this way Viel et al. (2000) demonstrate clustering of cases of soft-tissue sarcomas and non-Hodgkin's lymphomas, but not of Hodgkin's disease, around a solid-waste incinerator with high emission levels of dioxin in France. The authors conclude that further studies would be needed to confirm the relationship between dioxin exposure and soft-tissue sarcoma and non-Hodgkin's lymphoma risk. In two recent applications the focused spatial scan statistic has been used to link BSE cases to specific feed mills. Using a number of models, Sheridan et al. (2005) confirm spatio-temporal clustering of cattle herds in Ireland (1996–2000). The spatial component is dominant and a focused test identifies high-risk feed mills at the centroids of clusters. Schwermer et al. (2007), investigating BSE cases in Switzerland (1996–2001), use as cluster centres the locations of feed producers that tested positive for contamination of cattle feed with meat and bone meal. They conclude that whilst a causal link is suggested by their results, other factors must also play a part since BSE clusters occurred around only some producers of contaminated feed.

A particularly innovative application of the focused spatial scan statistic is its use to establish the origins of a *Trypanosoma brucei rhodesiense* sleeping sickness outbreak in the Sorroti area of eastern Uganda. In an 18-month observational study, following an outbreak of sleeping sickness in Sorroti, Fevre et al. (2001) find that over half the cattle traded at the Brookes Corner cattle market originated from endemic sleeping sickness areas. A subsequent case-control study identifies distance to the cattle market as a highly significant risk factor for sleeping sickness, and by using the focused spatial scan statistic they demonstrate significant clustering of cases close to the market at the start of the outbreak. Software for implementing the focused spatial scan statistic includes SaTScan, the Dcluster package in R, and ClusterSeer.

5.5 Space–time cluster detection

5.5.1 Kulldorff's space–time scan statistic

The spatial scan statistic has been adapted to look for clusters in space and time by extending the idea of a two-dimensional circular window to that of a cylinder passing through time. This has been applied, using the Poisson model, to explore brain cancer distribution in Los Alamos, a remote New Mexican community established in 1943 to provide a workforce to the Los Alamos National Laboratory, a nuclear research and design facility (Kulldorff et al. 1998a). Kulldorff (2001) proposes the prospective use of the space–time scan statistic, with repeated time periodic analysis, as part of a surveillance system to track active clusters of disease, for detecting the geographic location of emerging clusters and evaluating their significance. He demonstrates this with the Los Alamos data. In a later development of the original 'prospective space–time scan statistic' (Kulldorff 2001), Kulldorff et al. (2005) develop the 'space–time permutation scan statistic', which does not require

data on the background population at risk, but estimates expected disease occurrence based only on case data. They demonstrate this adaptation using daily diarrhoea surveillance data from hospital emergency departments in New York City between November 2001 and November 2002.

Hjalmars et al. (1999) use the space–time scan statistic to investigate clustering of childhood malignant brain tumours in Sweden, demonstrating an increase in rates of these cancers during the period 1973 to 1992, but find no evidence for clustering in space or time. Viel et al. (2000), using a Poisson model, explore space–time clustering of soft-tissue sarcomas, non-Hodgkin's lymphomas, and Hodgkin's disease, around a solid-waste incinerator in France. Smith et al. (2000) use a Bernoulli model to explore space–time clustering of anthrax strains in the Kruger National Park in South Africa. The spatial and temporal distributions of two genotypes indicate the anthrax epidemic foci to be independent of each other. Sheehan et al. (2000) find significant clustering of breast cancer in western Massachusetts, USA. Ward (2001) uses the space–time scan statistic (Poisson model) to investigate clustering of sheep blowfly strike, controlling for the effect of flock size and composition, the presence of fly strike control measures, and rainfall. Other, more recent examples of the space–time scan statistic include explorations of clustering in viral diseases of farmed fish (Knuesel et al. 2003), leptospirosis in dogs (Ward 2002), and different molecular subtypes of human listeriosis (Sauders et al. 2003).

In an investigation of outbreaks of acute respiratory disease in Norwegian cattle herds, Norström et al. (2000) compare the space–time scan statistic to both Knox's method and Jacquez's *k* nearest neighbour test. They find that all the methods identify significant space–time clusters, but highlight the disadvantage of the subjective selection of space and time thresholds in the Knox test, and the disadvantage, common to both the Knox test and to the Jacquez *k* nearest neighbours test, that they assume the population size does not change through time. The prospective space–time scan statistic does not make this assumption, it can accommodate confounding covariates in the analysis and moreover, it has the advantage in that it identifies the actual locations of space–time clusters.

Kleinman et al. (2005) investigate various adjustments to the space–time scan statistic to account for underlying spatial and temporal trends in diseases. They find that when adjusting for day of the week, month, holidays, and local history of disease, smaller numbers of clusters of lower respiratory complaints are found (2% of days) compared to when unadjusted census population data are used (26% of days). Other recent examples of the application of space–time scan statistics include Recuenco et al. (2007), who identify a number of significant space–time clusters of enzootic racoon rabies in New York State (1997–2003), Sheehan and De Chello (2005) who demonstrate clusters of high and low incidence of late-stage breast cancer in Massachusetts (1988–1997), and Jones et al. (2006) who use the prospective space–time scan statistic to reveal clustering of shigellosis in Chicago, in 2002. Software for implementing the space-time scan statistic includes SaTScan, the Dcluster package in R, and ClusterSeer.

5.5.2 Example of space–time cluster detection

The space–time permutation of Kulldorff's spatial scan statistic was applied to the British cattle TB data for the period 1986 to 1997. The Bernoulli model was used and all TB-breakdown herds were included as cases compared to 30% of control herds, with the maximum cluster size set to 5% of all points (mainly to facilitate comparison with other analyses performed using these settings). Table 5.2 provides details of the 12 space–time clusters of TB breakdowns that were located, and Fig. 5.6 illustrates some details of these clusters: (a) log likelihood ratio, (b) prevalence, and (c) duration.

The results of the analysis are dominated by two large and highly significant clusters; Cluster 1 (labelled in Fig. 5.6), with its centre in Gloucestershire, and Cluster 2 spanning the Devon/Cornwall boundary. Both were relatively long-lasting but Cluster 2 had a much lower prevalence over this time period illustrating the need to consider all characteristics of clusters when making comparisons.

The results from cluster analysis of individual years (Fig. 5.5) can thus be compared with a single analysis over the entire period (Fig. 5.6). The latter presents the results of the analysis in a more condensed form, but at the risk of missing some of the subtleties that can be seen by looking at individual years.

5.6 Conclusion

This chapter has explored a variety of methods by which spatial and spatio-temporal disease clusters

Table 5.2 Details of space–time clusters illustrated in Figure 5.6. For each cluster the area is given, the start and end date, LLR is the log likelihood ratio, P(999) is the significance level based on 999 Monte Carlo replications (hence the plateau at 0.001), RR is the relative risk (observed/expected), which is directly proportional to Prev., (the prevalence corrected for sampling) over the duration of the cluster

Cluster	Area (km²)	Start	End	LLR	P(999)	RR	Prev.
1	5,830	1992	1997	1,150,4	0.001	9.5	0.042
2	5,148	1989	1997	743.6	0.001	5.9	0.002
3	316	1991	1997	212.1	0.001	13.1	0.006
4	209	1993	1997	78.2	0.001	15.1	0.009
5	194	1997	1997	41.3	0.001	20.5	0.063
6	194	1989	1997	41.1	0.001	33.8	0.012
7	21	1987	1996	24.3	0.001	43.1	0.013
8	27	1987	1994	21.8	0.001	11.2	0.004
9	47	1995	1997	20.6	0.003	39.9	0.041
10	479	1997	1997	18.1	0.017	14.5	0.045
11	15	1990	1992	14.3	0.382	37.3	0.038
12	13	1987	1996	13.7	0.721	97.0	0.030

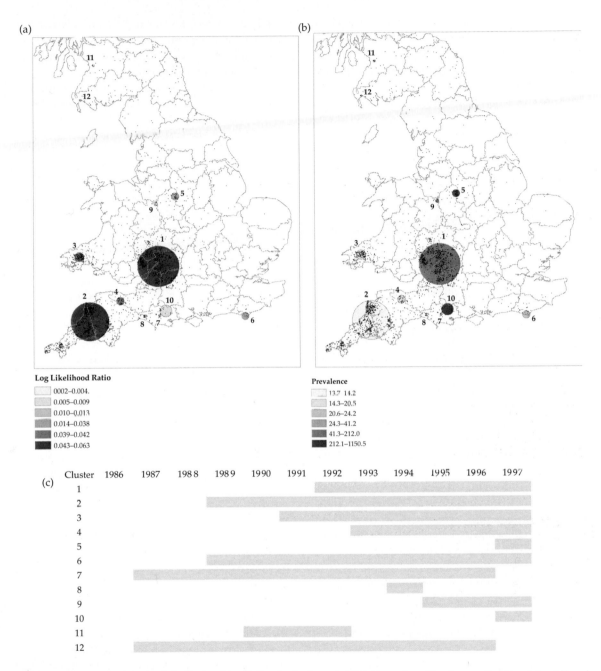

Figure 5.6 Space–time cluster analysis showing a) log likelihood ratios (i.e. probability), b) prevalence (directly proportional to relative risk), and c) duration of space–time clusters of TB breakdown herds in Britain from 1986 to 1977. Clusters were identified using the Bernoulli model of the space-time scan statistic with all TB breakdown herds as cases compared to 30% of control herds, with a maximum cluster size set to 5% of all points. See also Table 5.2.

can be identified statistically. New methods for detecting local clustering are continuously being developed. For example, Aamodt et al. (2006) compare the spatial scan statistic against a method based on generalized additive models (Hastie and Tibshirani 1991) and one using Bayesian approaches that have emerged from the Besag, York, and Mollié model (Besag et al. 1991). Other Bayesian approaches to cluster detection include those demonstrated by Neill et al. (2006) and Lawson (2006b), but these tend towards the modelling approaches that are described in detail in Chapters 6 and 7. Another recent advance is the development of a spatial hazard model for cluster detection (Gay et al. 2007), which can account for risk factors and for spatial heterogeneity in the population at risk. In terms of statistical methodology, the field of cluster detection is advancing rapidly.

A frequently quoted limitation common to many cluster detection tests (e.g. Besag and Newell (1991) and Cuzick and Edwards (1990)) is the *a priori* choice of cluster size, as testing for a variety of cluster sizes results in problems of multiple inference. Analysis of the British cattle TB data suggests this to be a central problem and there do not seem to be clear guidelines on how to deal with it.

Kulldorff et al. (1997) suggest, and demonstrate using an analysis of breast cancer in the northeast United States, a method of decomposing a significant cluster into non-overlapping sub-clusters, each of which would allow rejection of the null hypothesis on its own strength by sequentially limiting the maximum cluster size (the very approach adopted in Section 5.3.6). However, in the same paper he states that one of the reasons for the superiority of the spatial scan statistic over other cluster detection algorithms is that 'by searching for clusters without specifying their size or location, the method ameliorates the problem of pre-selection bias'.

Chaput et al. (2002), in a spatial analysis of HGE near Lyme, Connecticut, vary the maximum cluster size from 50 to 25% of the population at risk, in order to look for 'sub-clusters'. A large and highly significant cluster ($p = 0.001$) is identified at the 50% level, and with the 25% threshold two 'sub-clusters' emerged, one highly significant ($p = 0.001$) and the other considerably less so ($p = 0.16$). They argue that

by taking the default value of 50%, pre-selection bias is avoided and therefore the first analysis better represents the areas of increased risk for infection based on the spatial distribution of HGE in the area.

Jemal et al. (2002) report on the geographic analysis of prostate cancer mortality between 1970 and 1989 in the United States. They identify fairly large, significant clusters in a 'first round of analyses' and smaller sub-clusters in a 'second round of analyses'. Based on the very large size of a primary cluster of prostate cancer among white males in the northwest of the United States it must be assumed that they select 50% of the population as the upper limit. What is not clear is whether the sub-clusters are located by considering the clusters identified in the first round as independent populations (for new analyses), or by reducing the maximum cluster size (proportion of the population included) by some unspecified amount, in order to identify a larger number of smaller clusters (as was done in Section 5.3.6).

Boscoe et al. (2003) point out that those following Kulldorff's approach tend to select clusters with large areas containing large populations but only small elevations in disease risk, since these exhibit the highest levels of statistical power. Smaller areas, with lower levels of significance but higher prevalence or incidence rates, tend to be overlooked. They propose an adaptation to Kulldorff's approach that involves stratifying the set of statistically significant circles by relative risk. Within each risk stratum the non-overlapping circles with the highest likelihood are displayed in a nested manner. They demonstrate this method using prostate cancer mortality data from the USA.

As shown in Section 5.3.6 (specifically in Fig. 5.3), *a priori* choice of cluster size can have profound effects on the results. The grave concern arises that by exploring a range of maximum cluster sizes an upper cluster size threshold can be chosen that presents a pattern of clustering best suited to support a particular argument, rather than that which best reflects reality. This may cast doubt on the validity of the numerous studies that have been reported using scan circles, and in particular those based on the spatial scan statistic.

CHAPTER 6

Spatial variation in risk

6.1 Introduction

Whenever possible, epidemiological disease investigations should include an assessment of the spatial variation of disease risk, as this may provide important clues leading to causal explanations. The information presented may be, for example, the density of disease cases or spatial variation in an attribute value such as disease risk. The objective is to produce a map representation of the important spatial effects present in the data while simultaneously removing any distracting noise or extreme values. The resulting smoothed map should have increased precision without introducing significant bias (Haining 2003). The method used to analyse the data depends on how they have been recorded. If the data occur as point locations (e.g. outbreaks of disease) kernel smoothing methods can be applied to facilitate visual assessment of the pattern. In the case of data representing, for example, the incidence of infection within administrative areas, Bayesian methods can be applied to take account of the uncertainty of the local measurement and spatial dependence between neighbouring measurements. If the data represent sample point locations used to describe continuous fields, such as disease vector presence, interpolation methods such as kriging can be applied to generate spatially continuous representations.

6.2 Smoothing based on kernel functions

Visual analysis of point data density ranges from a simple display of locations to the use of smoothing methods for generating point density surface representations in raster format. In general, the first method should only be used if the number of points is limited so that different densities can still be differentiated visually. The map in Fig. 6.1a, showing the point locations of TB-infected herds, can be readily interpreted. However, Fig. 6.1b shows the point locations of all cattle herds TB-tested in Great Britain in 1996, and as a result of the large number of points it is not possible to differentiate between areas with high densities of points. In such situations, it is necessary either to generate estimates aggregated at some administrative level or to apply smoothing methods.

Spatial smoothing can be achieved by calculating simple localized averages or by applying more complex mathematical functions to the data. With both approaches a window, typically of fixed size, centres on each data point or polygon centroid. The degree of smoothing is influenced by the size and shape of the window (also called filter or kernel), as well as the mathematical function applied to the values within the window. The larger the window, the more information is 'borrowed' from the neighbouring areas, and the more statistically precise is the resulting smoothed estimate. The disadvantage is that in a spatially heterogeneous environment the estimates could be biased as they will be more strongly influenced by data values from locations some distance away (Burrough and McDonnell 1998; Haining 2003). As a consequence, important local clustering of increased or reduced point density may disappear in the kernel-smoothed representation. The results produced by spatial smoothing methods can also be biased by edge effects.

Spatial filters are applied in image enhancement to remove random noise, but are also available as a

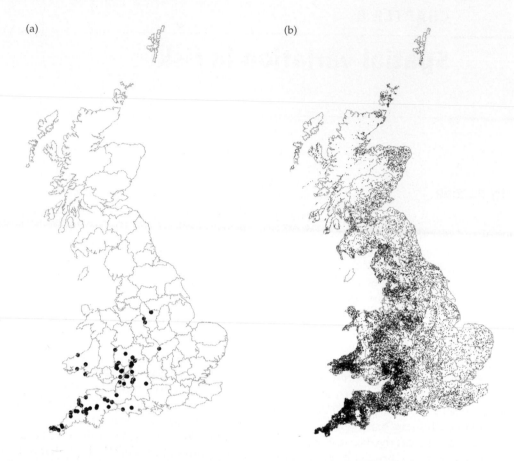

Figure 6.1 Point maps showing (a) the distribution of herds for which TB-positive cattle were identified at slaughter in 1996, and (b) locations of herds TB-tested in 1996, in Great Britain.

standard neighbourhood function in GIS (Bonham-Carter 1994). With epidemiological spatial data, they can be applied to point as well as aggregated data represented through a centroid. Talbot et al. (2000) describe the use of filters with fixed geographical size as well as with constant population size to generate smoothed map representations of disease ratios. They demonstrate that a filter with constant population size retains adequate spatial resolution in high density areas while at the same time producing stable rate estimates in low density areas.

Kernel density estimation is a special case of distance weighted map smoothing where a bivariate probability density function is applied to determine the intensity of a spatial point process (Bailey and Gatrell 1995). The following equation is used to perform the calculations:

$$\hat{\lambda}_\tau(s) = \frac{1}{\delta_\tau(s)} \sum_{i=1}^{n} \frac{1}{\tau^2} k\left(\frac{(s-s_i)}{\tau}\right) \tag{6.1}$$

where k() represents the chosen bivariate probability density function, $\tau > 0$ is the bandwidth, s is the point on which a disc of radius τ is centred, s_i are the points within the disc's area, and τ represents an edge correction factor. The difference between density and intensity should be noted, in that the former integrates to one and estimates are interpreted as probabilities, whereas the latter estimates the mean number of events per unit area and does not integrate to one. One can be converted into the other by a multiplicative constant.

The resulting smoothed density surface is influenced by the choice of probability density function,

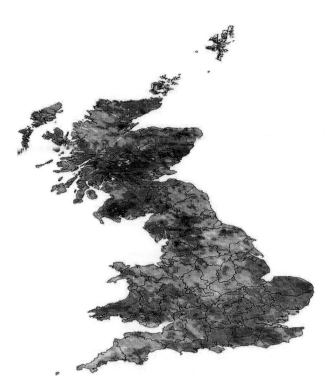

Plate 1 (Figure 1.3, page 8): False colour composite of Fourier-processed air temperature variables for Great Britain. The average value (the 'zero-order' component) is displayed in red, the phase of the first-order component is displayed in green, and the amplitude of the first-order component is displayed in blue.

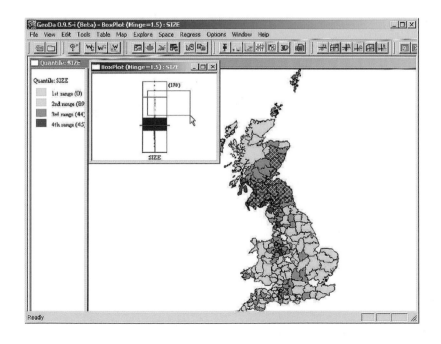

Plate 2 (Figure 3.5, page 21): Dynamic exploratory spatial data analysis (ESDA) using the GeoDa software. The screen shot shows two windows: (main) a choropleth map of area-level herd size, and (inset) a box-and-whisker plot showing the distributional features of the same data.

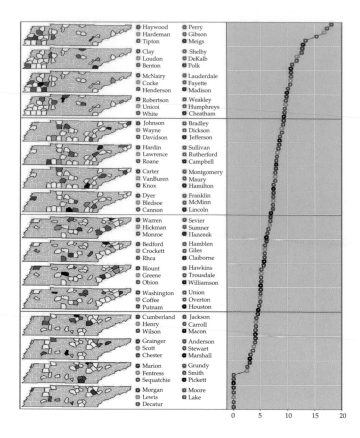

⊕ Haywood	⊕ Perry
⊕ Hardeman	⊕ Gibson
⊕ Tipton	⊕ Meigs
⊕ Clay	⊕ Shelby
⊕ Loudon	⊕ DeKalb
⊕ Benton	⊕ Polk
⊕ McNairy	⊕ Lauderdale
⊕ Cocke	⊕ Fayette
⊕ Henderson	⊕ Madison
⊕ Robertson	⊕ Weakley
⊕ Unicoi	⊕ Humphreys
⊕ White	⊕ Cheatham
⊕ Johnson	⊕ Bradley
⊕ Wayne	⊕ Dickson
⊕ Davidson	⊕ Jefferson
⊕ Hardin	⊕ Sullivan
⊕ Lawrence	⊕ Rutherford
⊕ Roane	⊕ Campbell
⊕ Carter	⊕ Montgomery
⊕ VanBuren	⊕ Maury
⊕ Knox	⊕ Hamilton
⊕ Dyer	⊕ Franklin
⊕ Bledsoe	⊕ McMinn
⊕ Cannon	⊕ Lincoln
⊕ Warren	⊕ Sevier
⊕ Hickman	⊕ Sumner
⊕ Monroe	⊕ Hancock
⊕ Bedford	⊕ Hamblen
⊕ Crockett	⊕ Giles
⊕ Rhea	⊕ Claiborne
⊕ Blount	⊕ Hawkins
⊕ Greene	⊕ Trousdale
⊕ Obion	⊕ Williamson
⊕ Washington	⊕ Union
⊕ Coffee	⊕ Overton
⊕ Putnam	⊕ Houston
⊕ Cumberland	⊕ Jackson
⊕ Henry	⊕ Carroll
⊕ Wilson	⊕ Macon
⊕ Grainger	⊕ Anderson
⊕ Scott	⊕ Stewart
⊕ Chester	⊕ Marshall
⊕ Marion	⊕ Grundy
⊕ Fentress	⊕ Smith
⊕ Sequatchie	⊕ Pickett
⊕ Morgan	⊕ Moore
⊕ Lewis	⊕ Lake
⊕ Decatur	

Plate 3 (Figure 3.6, page 22): Conditioned choropleth map of median infant mortality rate per 1000 births in the state of Tennessee, USA between 1992 and 1997. Reproduced from Carr et al. (2000) with permission from *Statistics in Medicine*.

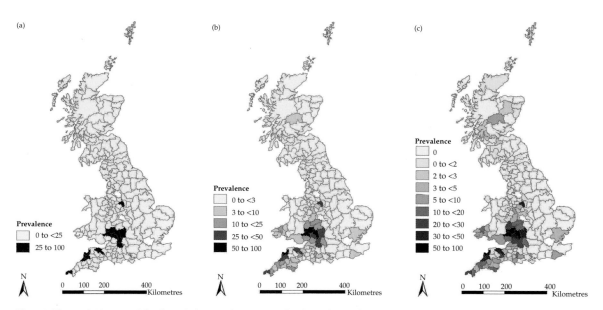

Plate 4 (Figure 3.10, page 29): Choropleth maps showing area-level prevalence of TB on British cattle holdings (expressed as the number of TB-positive holdings per 100,000 holdings) for 1985–1997 plotted using (a) two, (b) five, and (c) nine cutpoints.

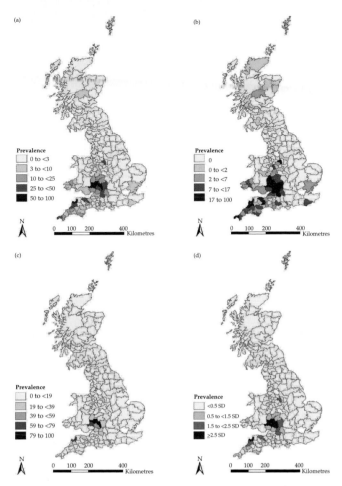

Plate 5 (Figure 3.11, page 30): Choropleth maps showing area-level prevalence of TB on British cattle holdings (expressed as the number of TB-positive holdings per 100,000 holdings) for 1985–1997 using (a) natural breaks, (b) quintile breaks, (c) equal interval breaks, and (d) standard deviation classifications.

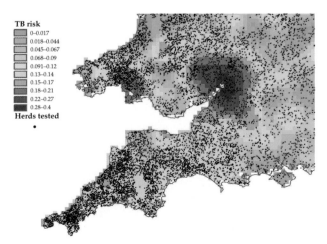

Plate 6 (Figure 6.3, page 72): Kernel density ratio surface for the southwest of England showing the risk of cattle herds testing positive for TB during 1996 (the locations of all herds tested are shown as black dots).

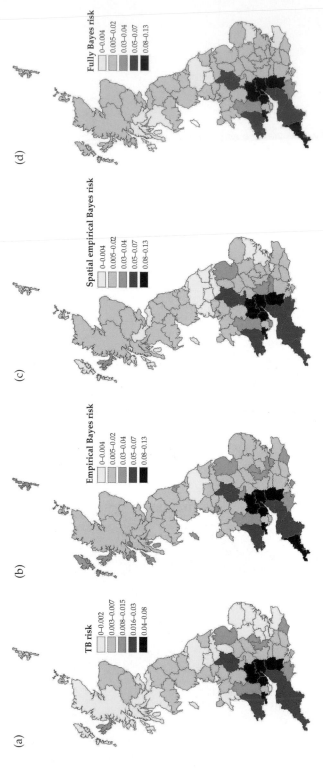

Plate 7 (Figure 6.4, page 74): Choropleth maps of TB-test results for cattle herds in Great Britian in 1999 aggregated by county. (a) Prevalence of TB-test positive cattle herds, (b) empirical Bayes risk of TB-test positive herds, (c) spatial empirical Bayes risk of TB-test positive herds, (d) fully Bayes risk of TB-test positive herds.

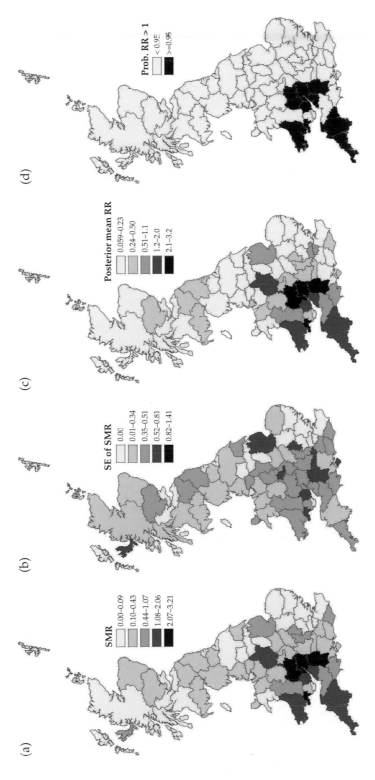

Plate 8 (Figure 6.5, page 75): Choropeth maps of standardized morbidity ratios (SMR) and Bayesian relative risk estimates for TB herd test results for cattle in Great Britain in 1999 aggregated by county, (a) SMR comparing TB reactor risk between counties, (b) standard error of SMR, (c) fully Bayesian estimates of relative risk of TB-test reactor herds, and (d) statistically significant fully Bayesian relative risks of reactor herds.

Prob. RR > 1
< 0.95
>=0.95

Posterior mean RR
0.059–0.23
0.24–0.50
0.51–1.1
1.2–2.0
2.1–3.2

SE of SMR
0.00
0.01–0.34
0.35–0.51
0.52–0.81
0.82–1.41

SMR
0.00–0.09
0.10–0.43
0.44–1.07
1.08–2.06
2.07–3.21

(a)

(b)

(c)

(d)

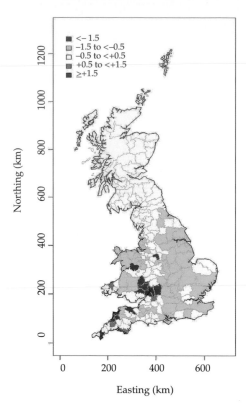

Plate 9 (Figure 7.6, page 91): Choropleth map showing the spatial distribution of the area-level standardized residuals from the fixed-effects Poisson model of area-level TB risk in Great Britain shown in Table 7.2.

Plate 10 (Figure 7.14, page 108): Mean (of 100) posterior probability risk map of bovine tuberculosis (TB) cases in Great Britain predicted by discriminant analytical models using step-wise inclusion of 10 variables to maximize the area under the curve (AUC) at each step. Five presence and five absence clusters were used for each bootstrap sample of 300 presence and 300 absence points sampled at random, with replacements, from a population of 482 presence and 3000 absence pixels (a presence pixel is a 0.01 degree pixel with at least one TB-positive farm in 1997; an absence pixel has farms, but no TB-positive ones in the same period). Posterior probability is on the green to red colour scale shown in the legend beneath the figure. The positive pixels are indicated by the black dots.

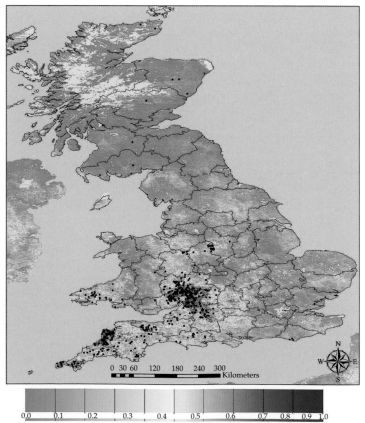

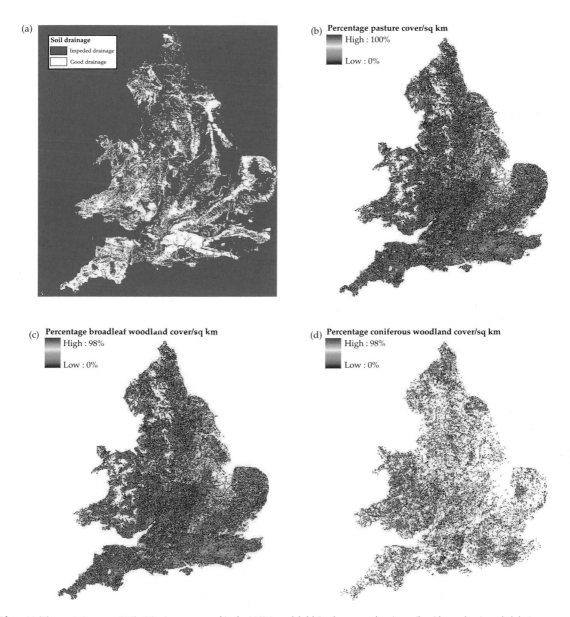

Plate 11 (Figure 8.2, page 116): Criterion maps used in the MCDA model. (a) Boolean map showing soils with good or impeded drainage, (b) a continuous scale map of pasture in England and Wales (percentage cover/km²), (c) a continuous scale map of broadleaf woodland in England and Wales (percentage cover/km²), and (d) a continuous scale map of coniferous woodland in England and Wales (percentage cover/km²).

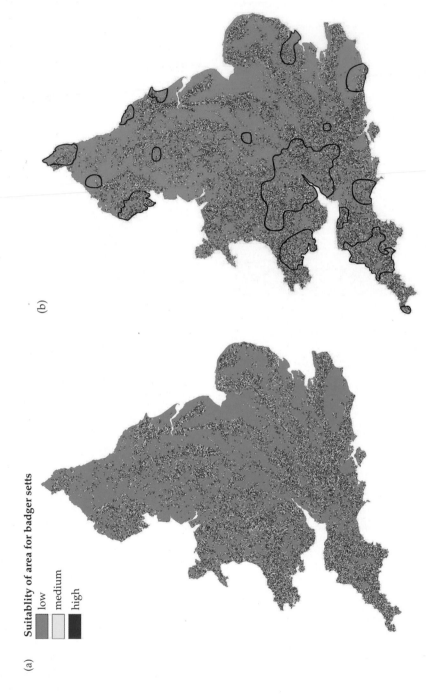

(a)

Suitablity of area for badger setts

low

medium

high

(b)

Plate 12 (Figure 8.3, page 117): (a) Map identifying areas in England and Wales of low, medium, and high suitability for the construction of badger setts, and (b) the suitability map with an overlay of the 1996 TB high-risk areas in England and Wales.

bandwidth τ, and size of the grid cells for each of which an individual density estimate is calculated. The mathematical function used to define the kernel specifies the pattern for down-weighting the influence of points further away from the point locations for which intensity is to be estimated. Different mathematical functions can be used but they are considered to have less influence on the estimation than the bandwidth, and the Gaussian kernel is therefore often used for the sake of computational simplicity (Waller and Gotway 2004). The latter is the width of the kernel function and therefore determines the distance over which points will be included in the calculation, and the larger it is the smoother the resulting surface. The bandwidth τ can be obtained using mathematical calculations or by subjective choice. Haining (2003) emphasizes that it is not about obtaining an optimal bandwidth based on theoretical considerations, but rather about generating a spatially smoothed surface that reveals insights into the underlying data. Characteristics of the biological process to be studied could therefore be used to guide the choice, and it is always recommended to explore surfaces generated by different bandwidth estimates. Diggle (2003) recommends that, rather than an automatic procedure, a plot of the mean square error of the non-parametric intensity estimator against different values of τ be used to inform the choice of bandwidth. Adaptive bandwidth selection methods vary the local bandwidth during the estimation process so that a minimum number of observations are included (Bailey and Gatrell 1995). Further details and discussions in relation to bandwidth selection methods can be found in Scott (1992) and Wand and Jones (1995). The kernel density calculation method should also take account of edge effects (also called spatial censoring) to minimize the bias of estimations close to the boundary of the study area (Lawson et al. 1999b). This can be achieved, for example, by adjusting the area used in the calculation process according to the overlap of the circular area defined by the bandwidth and the study region (Diggle 2003). When using kernel density estimation functions built into GIS software products such as ArcGIS (ESRI, Redlands, California, USA) the bivariate Gaussian kernel is typically used, a

default algorithm is applied to calculate the bandwidth and no correction is made for edge effects. ArcGIS calculates the bandwidth as the minimum dimension (x or y) of the extent of the point theme divided by 30. More sophisticated methods for applying kernel smoothing can be implemented using the statistical functions developed for the software R. Stevenson et al. (2000) conduct a descriptive spatial analysis of BSE occurrence in Great Britain using kernel density estimation based on a Gaussian kernel and a fixed bandwidth of 30 km, estimated using the normal optimal method described by Bowman and Azzalini (1997) and implemented in the SM library for R by the same authors. Choice of the grid cell size for which the kernel-smoothed intensity estimates are to be produced needs to be considered from a presentational, biological, and numerical perspective. Since the objective is to achieve a balance between producing a smooth surface while still describing the relevant spatial variation in intensity, grid cells that are too small needlessly increase the data storage required, and if too large may hide relevant patterns. It is therefore sensible to make the grid cells larger than the geographical extent of the biological unit of interest. For example, if the density of farms is to be estimated, the grid cell size should be larger than the area covered by an average farm. If the grid cell size is too small, the intensity estimates will be very small numbers that may be more difficult to interpret. As with the bandwidth, the algorithm implemented in the software may use default settings to define grid cell size that are often not 'optimal' for the particular dataset. Fig. 6.2a shows kernel smoothed presentations of the density of all British cattle herds TB-tested in 1996 and Fig. 6.2b shows those that tested positive. Both estimations were made using a grid cell size of 5 km and a bandwidth of 30 km. This choice was based on the following considerations: firstly, from a national decision-making perspective, variability between areas above 25 km^2 was considered to be the focus of the analysis and secondly, local herd density estimates should not be influenced by densities at a distance of more than 30 km whereas bandwidth estimates below that would result in too much variability to allow meaningful policy-relevant interpretation. These considerations were based to a large degree on subjective choices. Fig. 6.2b shows the spatial distribution of TB-test positive herds. In order to identify unusually high occurrences of these herds, the spatial distribution of the underlying population at risk (Fig. 6.2a) also needs to be considered. This is difficult to perform through visual comparison of the two maps.

As in the example presented above, the distribution of the population at risk is usually spatially heterogeneous and therefore, to be able to detect spatial clusters of unusually high or low case intensity, it is necessary to examine the spatial pattern of the proportionality between intensity of disease cases and non-cases, or population at risk (sum of cases and non-cases). This method has been called extraction mapping (Lawson and Williams 1993). If data on the intensity of the population at risk cannot be obtained, the spatial distribution of another disease can be used instead, as long as it is not subject to the same aetiological processes and there is no differential reporting bias (Lawson 2001b). The ratio between the intensity of cases and the population at risk becomes the log disease risk, whereas if the denominator represents the intensity of controls (=non-cases) it is interpreted as a log relative risk (Kelsall and Diggle 1995b). One requirement of such ratio calculations is that the denominator should not take on zero values, which means that the bivariate Gaussian kernel with its non-zero tail should be used. The optimal bandwidths chosen for producing the individual intensity surfaces may not be appropriate for generating the ratio surface. The resulting ratio surface is also much more sensitive to different choices of bandwidth than the individual surfaces. There is some debate as to whether the numerator and denominator in this calculation should be generated using the same or different bandwidths (Bithell 1990; Bailey and Gatrell 1995; Diggle 2000). The preference seems to be that it should be the same, even if the sample sizes differ between the two populations (Kelsall and Diggle 1995a). Schabenberger and Gotway (2005) describe a visual exploratory approach for choosing the appropriate bandwidth and size of grid cells, based mainly on balancing the resolution and stability of the estimates in the context

of their biological interpretation. The statistical precision of the ratio estimates can be quantified using Monte Carlo methods (Kelsall and Diggle 1995b). Kernel regression methods have been proposed by Kelsall and Diggle (1998) as an alternative to the density ratio method. An advantage of this approach is that covariates can be included in the analysis.

Fig. 6.2c shows the ratio of the intensity surfaces of TB-test positive and all cattle herds tested as part of routine herd testing in Great Britain in 1996. It illustrates that it can be difficult to obtain stable risk estimates if intensities vary substantially across an area, such as with cattle-herd density in Great Britain where, particularly in Scotland, high risks were calculated based on very small numbers of herds at risk. This could be prevented by increasing the grid cell size and/or bandwidth of the kernel-smoothed maps but at the expense of spatial differentiation in the main areas of interest, namely Wales and the southwest of England. Fig. 6.3 shows the southwest of England where the risk estimates provide an interesting insight into the spatial pattern of positive routine herd testing. Cornwall and Devon have a lower risk of herds testing positive than the areas within the counties of Gwent, Gloucestershire, Avon, and Hereford and Worcester. There are also small clusters of increased risk in the counties of Dyfed, Powys, and Somerset.

6.3 Smoothing based on Bayesian models

Statistics used in the spatial representation of aggregated (e.g. province or district-level) disease risk data include relative risk, and standardized mortality/morbidity ratios (SMR). The SMR is the classic statistic used in representing spatial patterns of disease distribution. It standardizes the data by re-expressing them as the ratio between the observed number of cases and the number that would have been expected in a standard population. At whatever level of spatial aggregation (i), for a specified time period:

$$SMR_i = y_i/e_i \qquad (6.2)$$

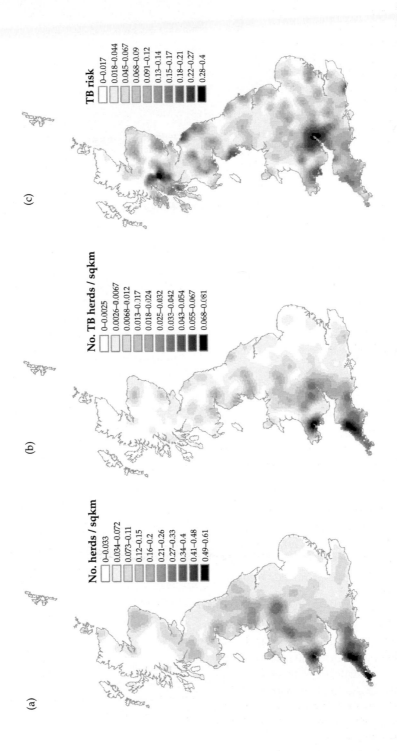

Figure 6.2 Kernel smoothed map representations of cattle herd densities in Great Britain. (a) Kernel smoothed intensity of **all** cattle herds tested using routine TB herd testing in 1995 (5 km grid cells, 30 km bandwidth), (b) kernel smoothed intensity of cattle herds tested **positive** during routine TB herd testing in 1996 (5 km grid cells, 30 km bandwidth), and (c) ratio of kernel smoothed intensities of test positive herds and all cattle herds tested in 1996.

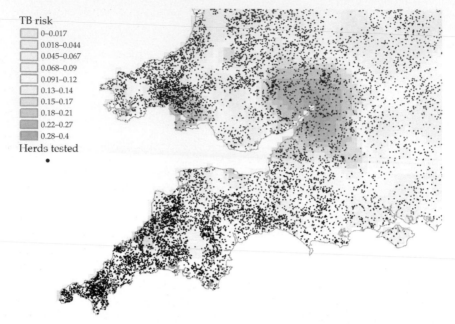

TB risk
- 0–0.017
- 0.018–0.044
- 0.045–0.067
- 0.068–0.09
- 0.091–0.12
- 0.13–0.14
- 0.15–0.17
- 0.18–0.21
- 0.22–0.27
- 0.28–0.4

Herds tested
•

Figure 6.3 Kernel density ratio surface for the southwest of England showing the risk of cattle herds testing positive for TB during 1996 (the locations of all herds tested are shown as black dots). See plate 6.

where y_i is the observed number of cases in area i, and the expected number of cases, e_i, is given by:

$$e_i = \frac{\sum y_i}{\sum n_i} \cdot n_i \qquad (6.3)$$

where n_i, is the observed population at risk in area i. National level disease risk or rate, for example, can be used to calculate the expected number of cases for each local area (Lawson and Williams 2001). The disadvantage of such SMR maps is that they tend to be dominated by areas with small numbers of observations, or if they focus on the statistical significance of the estimates, they tend to be dominated by areas with large populations, but potentially less important disease occurrence (Leyland and Davies 2005).

Clayton and Kaldor (1987) recognize that empirical Bayes methods can be used to generate maps that make use of the neighbourhood relationships in the data to produce statistically more precise risk estimates. Fully Bayesian estimation methods have been made possible through the development of the Markov Chain Monte Carlo (MCMC) algorithm, based on the Gibbs sampler (a special case of the Metropolis–Hastings algorithm; Gelman et al. 1995).

The basic principle of Bayesian methods is that uncertain data can be strengthened by combining them with prior information. In the case of empirical Bayes estimation of spatially-varying disease risk, posterior risk can be estimated from a weighted combination of the local risk (also called the likelihood) and the risk in surrounding areas, the latter representing the prior information (Clayton and Bernardinelli 1992; Wakefield et al. 2000). The relative weights for the two components depend on the sample size in the local area. If the local population size is large it will receive a strong weighting in the calculation process. If it is relatively small, its weighting is reduced and the derived estimate will tend towards the prior. The risk can be smoothed using a prior based on the global mean or on summarized data from the neighbouring areas. The smoothed risk is more stable and has higher specificity. It is recognized that Bayesian estimation always represents a trade-off between improved precision and the introduction of bias (Best et al. 2005).

The following formula is used to perform empirical Bayes calculations of disease risk (Bailey and Gatrell 1995):

$$\hat{\theta}_i = w_i r_i + (1 - w_i)\gamma_i \qquad (6.4)$$

where θ_i is the empirical Bayes estimate for area i, w_i are the weights applied to the local and neighbourhood estimates, r_i is the local risk in area i and γ_i is the mean of the prior, and r_i is the local risk in area i.

$$r_i = \frac{y_i}{n_i} \tag{6.5}$$

where y_i is the number of cases and n_i the population at risk in area i. The weights, w_i, in (6.4) are estimated as:

$$w_i = \frac{\phi_i}{(\phi_i + \gamma_i / n_i)} \tag{6.6}$$

where Φ_i is the variance of the prior, γ_i is the mean of the prior, and n_i the population at risk in area i.

The empirical Bayes prior specified above is purely spatial and is defined using the hyperparameters γ_i and Φ_i. The estimation is made by simplified posterior distributions through likelihood or integral approximations (Lawson et al. 2003). In fully Bayesian estimation, the hyperparameters have hyperprior distributions resulting in the estimates for each area better approximating the true value. Empirical estimates conversely, are inexact and tend to oversmooth towards the global mean. In addition, fully Bayesian methods generate credibility intervals for each local estimate. It is also possible to have a hierarchical or multilevel structure to the prior. Besag et al. (1991) developed the convolution prior which consists of an unstructured and a structured spatial component. Parameter distributions are estimated using MCMC spatial modelling. This method involves taking very large numbers of samples from the posterior distributions of model parameters. Sampling based on the Gibbs sampler is performed using a Markov Chain where successive samples are dependent on each other. A key issue with MCMC modelling is to decide when to finish sampling (i.e. when posterior distributions of the various parameters have converged). Detailed introductions to Bayesian spatial analysis can be found in Lawson et al. (2003), Banerjee et al. (2004), and Congdon (2003). Chapter 7 explores Bayesian approaches in the context of identifying risk factors associated with disease.

Fig. 6.4a is a choropleth map showing the proportion of TB-positive cattle herds per county in Great Britain in 1999. While this type of map is easy to interpret it has the disadvantage that the size of the districts and the position of their boundaries is typically a reflection of administrative requirements rather than of the spatial distribution of epidemiological factors. Fig. 6.4b shows a map generated using empirical Bayes estimation with the prior being the national level herd infection prevalence. Fig. 6.4c employed a neighbourhood empirical Bayes approach where the local estimate has shrunk towards the mean prevalence estimates of the neighbouring counties. The fully Bayesian approach based on a convolution prior was used to generate the map in Fig. 6.4d (Besag et al. 1991). Examining the four different maps shows that some of the counties have quite different risk levels, when considering prior information. While most of the high risk areas (around Gloucestershire) remain consistent, Cornwall is only in the highest risk category when using empirical non-spatial or fully Bayes estimation. An alternative approach for assessing these data would be to focus on the differences between the counties and the national average. Fig. 6.5a presents SMR estimates for TB-infected herds aggregated at county level. As with the prevalence map (Fig. 6.4a), this is largely a function of sample size and it is therefore appropriate to accompany the map with a presentation of the variability of the estimates, such as in Fig. 6.5b. Fig. 6.5c shows the posterior mean relative risks for each county based on fully Bayesian estimation. The proportion of estimates with a relative risk of greater than one is presented in Fig. 6.5d. It identifies three groupings of counties with an elevated risk of TB-infected herds relative to the rest of the country.

6.4 Spatial interpolation

Spatially continuous surfaces for attribute values, such as risk of disease vector presence or environmental exposure variables, are often produced from data collected at a sample of spatially distributed sites. These could be, for example, traps for capturing the *Culicoides* midges that transmit the bluetongue virus, or epidemiological field surveys

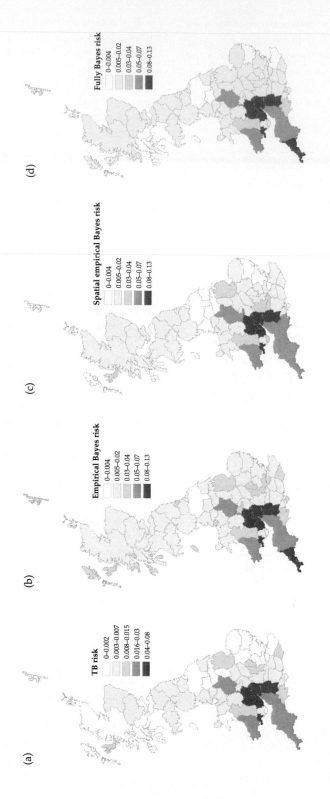

Figure 6.4 Choropleth maps of TB-test results for cattle herds in Great Britian in 1999 aggregated by county. (a) Prevalence of T3-test positive cattle herds, (b) empirical Bayes risk of TB-test positive herds, (c) spatial empirical Bayes risk of TB-test positive herds, (d) fully Bayes risk of TB-test positive herds. See plate 7.

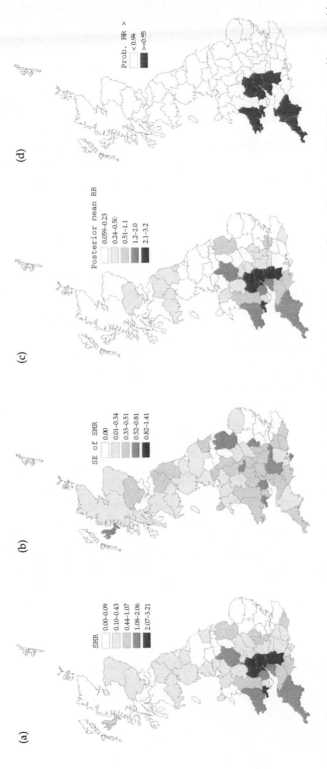

Figure 6.5 Choropeth maps of standardized morbidity ratios (SMR) and Bayesian relative risk estimates for TB herd test results for cattle in Great Britain in 1999 aggregated by county. (a) SMR comparing TB reactor risk between counties, (b) standard error of SMR, (c) fully Bayesian estimates of relative risk of TB-test reactor herds, and (d) statistically significant fully Bayesian relative risks of reactor herds. See plate 8.

that determine disease prevalence or incidence in a sample of herds or communities. Many environmental exposure variables describing, for example, water or air quality are measured at particular monitoring stations, but represent a spatially continuous phenomenon. One specific characteristic of this type of data is that its locations are fixed and known, and not random as is the case with the cluster analyses described in Chapters 4 and 5. Several methods can be used to convert these point location data into surface information. The simplest is to assign to each sampling point a polygon including all the hypothetically possible point locations that are closest to the sampling point. Dirichlet or Thiessen polygons fulfil this purpose but have the disadvantage that the resulting surface is discontinuous. The inverse distance weighting (IDW) interpolation method generates a continuous surface by calculating missing values from distance-weighted sample measurements. This method can be biased by the presence of local clusters. Kriging has the advantage in that it allows the errors of the imputed values to be estimated (Haining 2003). It can do this by not only accounting for the actual sample measurement values and their distance to the location to be predicted, but by also incorporating a mathematical model of the spatial dependence amongst sample measurements. Kriging was originally developed to describe continuous-scale outcome variables, such as the concentration of particular metals in the soil. Its use for non-Gaussian-type variables has been explored by several authors (Carrat and Valleron 1992; Webster et al. 1994; Diggle and Tawn 1998; Berke 2004; Graham et al. 2005; Goovaerts 2006). Stationarity is an important assumption of kriging (Bailey and Gatrell 1995; Graham et al. 2005), which means that the spatial correlation structure should be constant across locations. Typically however, this is not the case with data on disease counts, rates, and risks (Gotway and Wolfinger 2003), but the same authors conclude that, despite non-stationarity, mis-specified variogram functions, and assumptions of linear models for rate and count data, kriging estimates are relatively unbiased. The validity of using data aggregated to an area, such as in the case of disease frequency estimates per county, for producing point estimates using kriging has been confirmed by Kyriakidis (2004) and discussed further by Goovaerts (2006).

The basic model for interpolating a surface is based on the following equation (Waller and Gotway 2004):

$$\hat{Z}(s_0) = \sum_{i=1}^{N} \lambda_i Z(s_i) \qquad (6.7)$$

where $Z(s_i)$ is the measured value at the ith location, λ_i is the weight attributed to the measured value at the ith location, and s_0 is the prediction location.

This formula is used for both the IDW and kriging interpolation procedures, but they use different methods to calculate λ_i. With IDW it depends only on the distance to the prediction location whereas with kriging it is determined by the semivariogram, the distance to the prediction location and the spatial relationships between measurements around the prediction location. The empirical semivariogram shows the spatial dependence in the variable of interest as a scatterplot. Distance (spatial lag) is presented on the x- and semivariance on the y-axis. The semivariance is calculated as follows:

$$\hat{\gamma}(h) = \frac{1}{2|N(h)|} \sum_{N(h)} \left[Z(s_i) - Z(s_j) \right]^2 \qquad (6.8)$$

where $N(h)$ is the set of distinct pairs of values separated by h, $|N(h)|$ is the number of distinct pairs in $N(h)$.

The semivariogram can also be expressed as a covariance function but use of the former is preferred in spatial analysis. Schabenberger and Gotway (2005) provide a more detailed discussion of the relationship. The formula above describes a stationary and isotropic empirical semivariogram. If a spatial process is anisotropic, that is the spatial dependence varies with direction, different semivariograms can be estimated for each direction. Plotting the semi-variance produces a curve typically rising from a point on the y-axis (the nugget), to a maximum semi-variance value or 'sill' within a certain lag distance on the x-axis (the range) (see Fig. 6.6). The nugget describes the spatially uncorrelated variation or noise in the data. The larger this value the less spatial dependence there is amongst the attribute values and the less useful kriging interpolation will be. To provide a useful representation

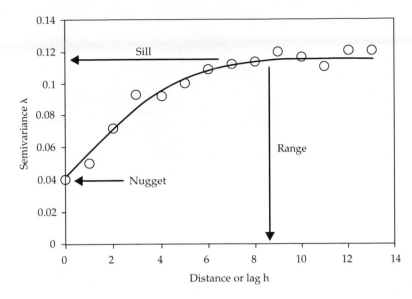

Figure 6.6 An empirical (circles) and theoretical (curve) semi-variogram

of the correlation structure, semi-variance should be calculated for about 10 to 20 lags with a maximum lag distance of about half the maximum separation distance between points (Waller and Gotway 2004; Schabenberger and Gotway 2005). (See Chapter 4 for an explanation of the difference between a semivariogram and a correlogram.)

Apart from providing information for kriging, the empirical semivariogram can be used as a generic tool for visually assessing the presence of spatial dependence or autocorrelation in a continuous process. This can also be useful for testing the assumption of independence for the residuals generated by a regression model. The empirical semivariogram cannot be used directly for kriging. Instead, a mathematical function has to be fitted to the curve, resulting in a theoretical semivariogram function that can then be used in the kriging process. The function can be derived from the variogram using statistical fitting algorithms or by visual assessment of the fit of standard mathematical functions. A flat shape of the resulting theoretical variogram function would suggest absence of spatial dependence. A function with, for example, an exponential shape with values increasing with distance reflects the presence of spatial dependence. Graham et al. (2005) use the shape of the semivariogram to draw conclusions about the relative

importance of spatial dependence and local herd effects on *Salmonella enterica* herd antibody levels.

Universal kriging can be used for non-stationary data, as it combines trend surface analysis and ordinary kriging into a single analysis. Amongst the various types of kriging, indicator, and co-kriging have been used to estimate disease risk surfaces. Indicator kriging models the probability of an event of interest. This could be, for example, the probability of an environmental contaminant being above a certain threshold level and is derived from input indicator data that needs to be in a binary format (zero indicating absence of, and one indicating presence of, the characteristic). The associated kriging variance reflects the uncertainty associated with the generated probability surface resulting from the interpolation process. Valencia et al. (2005) use this approach to predict the risk of ascariasis in children in Brazil. They report that they were able to improve the prediction by using co-kriging, which considered multiple covariates. Count data are interpolated by Ali et al. (2006) using Poisson kriging and Banerjee et al. (2004) describe Bayesian approaches to kriging. A more complete discussion of different kriging methods is provided in Waller and Gotway (2004).

Fig. 6.7b shows an example where ordinary kriging was used to generate a continuous surface

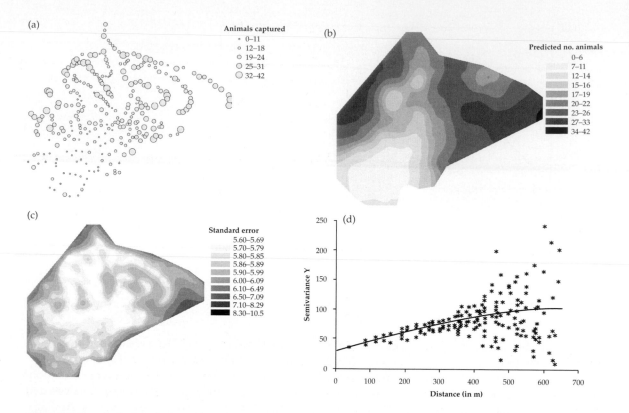

Figure 6.7 Example of ordinary kriging used to generate a continuous surface showing wild possum density in New Zealand derived from possum trap capture data. (a) Point map of trap locations with circle radius representing number of animals captured, (b) kriging surface map of predicted possum numbers, (c) standard error map for kriging estimates, and (d) semivariogram including model used to generate kriging surface.

of wild possum numbers based on trap-capture data for a study area (Fig. 6.7a). There were several problems associated with applying this technique to this particular dataset. Firstly, the traps did not cover the study area evenly and secondly, the data contained biological edge effects since the traps on the boundary would have attracted possums from outside the study area. The theoretical semivariogram function is based on fairly stable empirical semi-variance estimates up to a distance of 400m between point locations (Fig. 6.7d). No directional effects were detected when performing a directional semivariogram analysis using a semivariogram surface (not shown here). The standard error map (Fig. 6.7c) suggests that the error was relatively evenly distributed across the study area,

but increased towards the edge. In this particular case, kriging interpolation improved upon the information shown in the point map, resulting in a better impression of the variation in animal density across space. It does however need to be emphasized that, due to the data limitations described above, the predicted surface should only be used for broad interpretation of the underlying spatial variation in possum density.

Universal kriging has been applied in the example presented in Fig. 6.8 (which is presented in more detail in Berke (2004)). The semivariogram was fitted to tapeworm infection data in foxes, which were surveyed in Lower Saxony, Germany, between 1991 and 1997, aggregated at the level of 43 administrative regions. The choropleth map

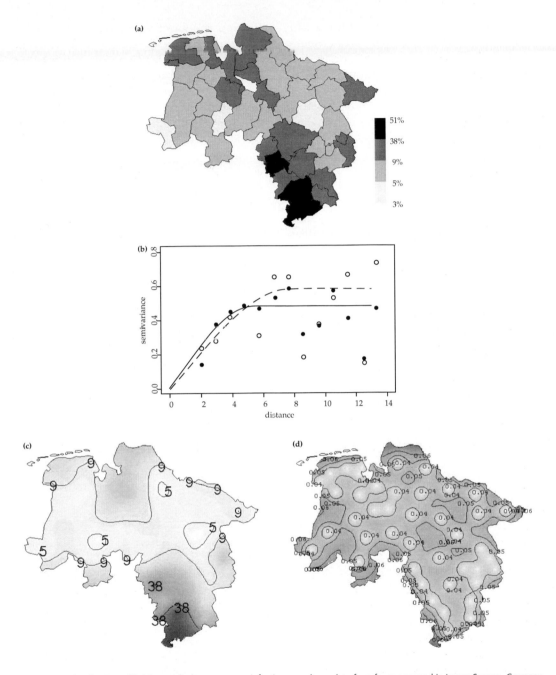

Figure 6.8 Example of universal kriging applied to tapeworm infection prevalence data from foxes surveyed in Lower Saxony, Germany (Reproduced with permission from Berke (2004)). (a) Choropleth map of empirical Bayes smoothed tapeworm prevalences, (b) empirical and theoretical semi-variogram detrended (solid line) and trend-contaminated (broken line) smoothed prevalences, (c) isopleth map from kriging smoothed prevalences, and (d) isopleth error map based on universal kriging standard errors.

shown in Fig. 6.8a indicates a spatial trend with prevalence levels increasing from north to south. Since this reflects the presence of non-stationarity, it is recommended to use universal rather than ordinary kriging. The spherical semivariogram functions shown in Fig. 6.8b demonstrate the benefit obtained from detrending the data, in that the sill is reduced. The resulting kriging surface shown in Fig. 6.8c maintains the key patterns shown in the choropleth map but avoids the jumps between regions. It also provides a prediction for the central Bremen region which had a missing value. The error map shown in Fig. 6.8d suggests the presence of a particular spatial pattern for the errors, which increases confidence in the validity of the model.

6.5 Conclusion

The presentation of spatial variation in risk is one of the most important functions of spatial analysis. If data have been collected for point locations or areas, enhanced visualization is possible by producing continuous surfaces using kernel smoothing and kriging interpolation. Both techniques are now available in most GIS software packages.

Kriging is subject to computational constraints when using large datasets as it assesses the co-variation between location pairs. While both methods can be used to produce a risk surface, there is otherwise only a limited degree of overlap with respect to suitable applications of the two methods. Kernel smoothing is subject to less restrictive statistical assumptions than kriging, and will not generate negative estimates for risk data. With aggregated ratio data, the statistical uncertainty of local risk estimates can elegantly be reduced by taking advantage of spatial dependence through Bayesian methods. If further smoothing is considered desirable, the Bayesian area estimates can be converted into a smooth surface using kriging. All these methods however, result in changes to the original data values. While this should result in improvements with respect to visual interpretation, it is also likely that artefacts and biases will be introduced and particular care needs to be taken in order to minimize these. Rather than being able to rely solely on the statistical methods, in most cases the user is required to make decisions about the parameters needed for the smoothing algorithms, and these subjective decisions may have quite a dramatic effect on the outcome.

CHAPTER 7

Identifying factors associated with the spatial distribution of disease

7.1 Introduction

The concepts and techniques discussed so far have dealt with describing, visualizing, and exploring spatial data. In this chapter the analytical techniques of regression and discrimination are introduced as a means of quantifying the effect of a set of explanatory variables on the spatial distribution of a particular outcome. The material presented here is similar to that which might be presented in standard statistical texts, but includes an overview of the modifications needed to account for the spatial dependency frequently associated with disease data.

Perhaps the first aspect to consider is the type of outcome variable under investigation. In epidemiology interest lies in understanding patterns of disease in populations, so it is often the case that the outcome variable is either a count of disease events for area units (see for example Jarup et al. 2002), or more simply a binary response indicating the presence or absence of disease at a given location (see for example Diggle et al. 2002). Less frequently in epidemiology (compared with other disciplines) outcomes may be measured on a continuous scale, for example, concentrations of carbon monoxide in an urban environment (Best et al. 2000). Knowledge of the type of outcome variable is important since it determines the regression technique to be used and the options available to account for spatial dependence.

This chapter is divided into four sections. The first outlines the principles of linear, Poisson, and logistic regression in order to provide a background to the material presented later in the chapter. The second section discusses the options available to

identify and account for spatial dependency in data when modelling. The third section reviews the common analytical techniques available for dealing with the three major spatial data types (area, point, and continuous data), and the fourth deals with discriminant analysis. The aim is to provide a broad overview of the available methodologies, highlighting the additional information to be gained by accounting for spatial dependence, and to suggest ways in which this information might be used to better understand the determinants of disease in human and animal populations. For a more in-depth discussion the reader is directed to the references cited in each section of the text. Throughout, the British cattle TB data are used to illustrate the concepts discussed.

7.2 Principles of regression modelling

7.2.1 Linear regression

Linear regression allows the mean value of a continuous outcome variable (also known as a response or dependent variable) μ_i to be represented as a function of m explanatory (also known as covariate, predictor, or independent) variables:

$$\mu_i = \beta_0 + \beta_1 X_{1i} + \ldots + \beta_m X_{mi} + \varepsilon_i \tag{7.1}$$

If the term X is used to represent the ($m \times i$) matrix of explanatory variables, the term β_0 in (7.1) is a constant indicating the value of μ_i when $X = 0$. The constants $\beta_1, \ldots, \beta_m$ determine how much the outcome variable changes in response to unit changes in each of the m explanatory variables.

Linear regression is a technique that can be used to model the broad-scale (first-order) spatial trend of a dataset where the outcome variable is continuously distributed. If data locations are represented by easting and northing coordinates (x_i and y_i), we can model the mean of the outcome variable μ_i as a function of location:

$$\mu_i = \beta_0 + \beta_1 x_i + \beta_2 y_i + \varepsilon_i \qquad (7.2)$$

(7.2) specifies a tilted plane for the spatial trend in μ with the amount of tilt dependent on the estimated values of β_0, β_1, and β_2. Extending the model to include quadratic terms, for example:

$$\mu_i = \beta_0 + \beta_1 x_i + \beta_2 x_i^2 + \beta_3 x_i y_i + \beta_4 y_i + \beta_5 y_i^2 + \varepsilon_i \quad (7.3)$$

allows the spatial trend to be non-linear. Note the following key assumptions behind this type of regression analysis:

1. For all values of μ there must be a corresponding value of X (the assumption of existence).
2. The value of μ at any point is not affected by the value of μ at any other point (independence).
3. The relationship between μ and X should be approximately linear (linearity).
4. The variance of μ about the estimated regression line is equal for all values of X (that is, the variance is said to be homoscedastic).
5. The residuals ε are normally distributed with a mean of zero (normality).

To illustrate, the British cattle TB data were used to develop a linear regression model of geographic and climatic factors influencing herd size. As some or all of the diet of British cattle is derived from pasture, the hypothesis might be that herd size is largest in those areas of the country where climatic conditions are suitable for pasture growth. To simplify the analysis, Great Britain was divided into 178 areas (after Stevenson et al. 2005) and median herd size calculated for each area. Similarly, area-level medians were calculated for each environmental variable relating to topography, temperature, water, and moisture. A standard model-building approach was then followed. The relationship between herd size and each of the 58 candidate explanatory variables was assessed using scatterplots and the Kruskal–Wallis test. Explanatory variables individually associated with herd size at an alpha level of less than 0.20 were included in a multivariate model. Using a backward-stepwise selection process, a two-tailed t test was applied to test the null hypothesis that each of the estimated regression coefficients was equal to zero. Variables with regression coefficients not significantly different from zero were removed from the model one at a time, beginning with the least significant, until the estimated regression coefficients for all retained explanatory variables were significant at the alpha level of 0.05. A check for collinearity was carried out by calculating the variance inflation factor for each variable (Armitage et al. 2002). The final model is shown in Table 7.1.

The results of this linear regression model show that median herd size is negatively associated with elevation and the maximum channel 3 amplitude (a measure of emitted thermal radiation and reflected light), and positively associated with maximum NDVI (a measure of vegetative activity) and the bi-annual amplitude of VPD (a measure of atmospheric dryness). The results indicate that median herd sizes are largest at low elevations, in areas of high vegetative activity, and where there

Table 7.1 Point estimates and standard errors of the regression coefficients in a multiple regression model of topography and climatic factors influencing the median size of cattle herds in 178 areas of Great Britian

Explanatory variable	Coefficient	SE	t	P-value
Intercept	−1,207.0	152.3	−7.92	<0.01
Elevation (metres above sea level)	−0.1121	0.0327	−3.43	<0.01
Max channel 3 amplitude (°K)	−0.9802	0.2540	−3.86	<0.01
Max NDVI	0.7524	0.0889	8.46	<0.01
Bi-annual VPD amplitude (mbar)	0.2141	0.0598	3.57	<0.01

NDVI: Normalized Difference Vegetation Index. VPD: Vapour pressure deficit.

is a large range in atmospheric dryness measured throughout the year. In short, these results are consistent with the observation that herd sizes are largest in those areas of the country that provide conditions suitable for pasture growth.

With a basic model developed the next step is to evaluate it for: (1) 'unusual' data (i.e. individual data points that do not show the same relationships as the bulk of the data), and (2) the distribution and pattern of variance in the error terms, and (3) non-linearity. The diagnostic plot series shown in Fig. 7.1 indicated that the residual terms were heteroscedastic; fitted values of greater than 60 show greater variation compared with the fitted values of 60 or less (Fig. 7.1a) and were not normally distributed (Fig. 7.1b). Applying the Breusch–Pagan test

(Breusch and Pagan 1979) to these data indicated that the observed heteroscedasticity was unlikely to have occurred by chance (Breusch–Pagan test statistic = 20.44; df = 4; p < 0.01). Lack of normality in the residuals (Fig. 7.1b) and lack of homogeneity in the variance of the residuals (Fig. 7.1a) represents violation of the assumptions of linear regression modelling, suggesting that the model should be reparameterized (see Section 7.6).

7.2.2 Poisson regression

When the outcome of interest is a count of the number of events occurring in a population of a given size, or a count of the number of events in relation to the number of person- or animal-years at risk, a

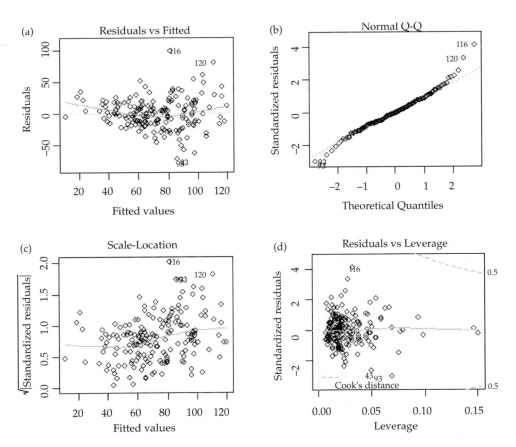

Figure 7.1 Regression diagnostics for the multiple linear regression model of median herd size in Great Britain. (a) Residuals versus fitted values, (b) normal Q-Q plot, (c) scale location plot, and (d) residuals versus leverage plot.

reasonable assumption is that these counts follow a Poisson distribution (especially for diseases that are either non-contagious or rare).

To illustrate the regression technique appropriate for Poisson-distributed data, the British cattle TB dataset was considered. For this analysis the total number of TB-positive holdings in each of the 178 previously-described areas of Great Britain was determined, and the area-level median calculated for each of the environmental variables included in the dataset. The aim of the analysis was to determine which of the environmental variables, if any, explained the variation in the number of TB-positive holdings in each area.

The area-level count of TB-positive holdings is presented in Fig. 7.2 and a frequency histogram of these data is shown in Fig. 7.3. Fig. 7.2 shows that number of TB-positive holdings is greatest in the southwest of England, southwest Wales, and parts of the Midlands. The frequency histogram of these data shows a skewed distribution with most areas reporting no TB-positive holdings and a small number of areas reporting greater than 40 TB-positive holdings.

Given the skewed distribution in Fig. 7.3 it is reasonable to assume that area-level counts of TB-positive holdings (O_i) follow a Poisson distribution. Furthermore, the observed area-level count is an estimate of the true number of TB-positive holdings in each area (μ_i), which is the product of exposure time in each area (n_i) and the incidence rate of disease (λ_i):

$$\mu_i = n_i \lambda_i \qquad (7.4)$$

The incidence rate of TB among holdings can be parameterized as a function of a series of m explanatory variables,

$$\log(\lambda_i) = (\beta_0 + \beta_1 X_{1i} + \ldots + \beta_m X_{mi}) + \varepsilon_i \qquad (7.5)$$

so that an estimate of the true number of TB-positive holdings in each area is given by:

$$\log(\mu_i) = \log(n_i) + (\beta_0 + \beta_1 x_{1i} + \ldots + \beta_m x_{mi}) + \varepsilon_i \qquad (7.6)$$

In (7.6) the term $\log(n_i)$ is an adjustment known as an *offset* which accounts for areas with different times at risk. If all areas had the same number of holdings and were observed for the same amount of time, the offset would not be required. In (7.6) the

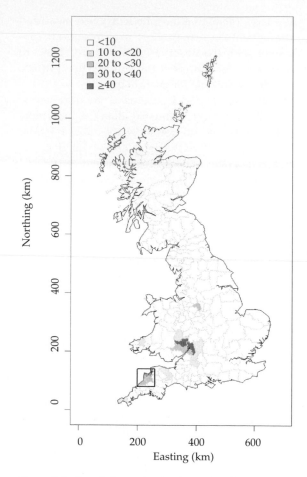

Figure 7.2 Choropleth map showing the number of TB-positive holdings in 178 areas of Great Britain. The boxed area shows the boundaries of the study area used for the logistic regression analyses described in Section 7.2.3.

terms $(\beta_0 + \beta_1 x_{1i} + \ldots + \beta_m x_{mi})$ represent an adjustment to account for disease counts that are either above or below that expected, based on time at risk. The error term, ε_i, represents a log-normal measure of the residual risk of disease in area i after accounting for each of the m explanatory variables.

Be aware that aggregating the data in this way may inadequately represent the exposure-response relationship at the individual holding level, an effect known as cross-level or ecological bias (Piantadosi et al. 1988; Plummer and Clayton 1996). However, the value of such analyses is to identify areas where the incidence of disease is not accounted for by known risk factors (i.e. the explanatory

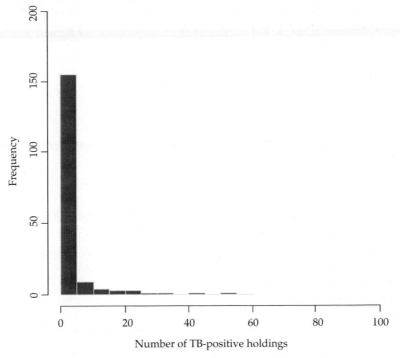

Figure 7.3 Frequency histogram showing the number of TB-positive holdings in 178 areas of Great Britain.

variables included in the model). These areas, once identified, might then be targeted for further investigative effort to establish, for example, if the unexplained excess (captured in the residual term) is uniformly or non-uniformly distributed across the individual units of interest.

A Poisson regression model of environmental factors influencing the count of TB-positive holdings in each of the 178 areas of Great Britain is described below. If O_i equals the number of TB-positive holdings in the ith area and n_i is the total number of holdings at risk in the ith area, the expected number of TB-positive holdings in each area is given by:

$$E_i = n_i \left(\frac{\sum\limits_{i=1}^{178} O_i}{\sum\limits_{i=1}^{178} n_i} \right) \tag{7.7}$$

The SMR for TB (i.e. the ratio of the observed number of TB-positive holdings to the number expected), can be compared with each of the explanatory variables using scatterplots and Spearman's rank correlation coefficients.

For parsimony, explanatory variables for area-level TB counts were restricted to those related to atmospheric dryness and environmental temperature. Similar to the approach used for developing the linear regression model described in Section 7.2.1, only those explanatory variables associated with area-level TB SMR at an alpha level of < 0.20 at the bivariate level were included in the model, and a backward-stepwise selection process was used to obtain the final model. A check for collinearity was performed by calculating the variance inflation factor for each variable in the final model. The regression coefficients in the final model are presented in Table 7.2 and show that area-level TB risk is positively associated with the annual phase of VPD, the annual phase of air temperature, and mean air temperature, but negatively associated with maximum air temperature.

As with the linear regression model (Section 7.2.1), the Poisson model was investigated for violation of any statistical assumptions using a series

Table 7.2 Point estimates and standard errors of regression coefficients in a fixed-effects Poisson regression model of climatic factors influencing area-level counts of TB-positive holdings in Great Britain

Explanatory variable	Coefficient	SE	z	P-value	RR (95% CI)
Intercept	−0.3551	0.0620	−5.72	<0.01	
Annual phase of VPD (mbar)	0.3032	0.0512	5.92	<0.01	1.35 (1.22−1.50)
Mean air temperature (°K)	0.0475	0.0065	7.33	<0.01	1.05 (1.04−1.06)
Maximum air temperature (°K)	−0.0127	0.0032	−3.91	<0.01	0.99 (0.98−0.99)
Annual phase of air temperature (°K)	0.0495	0.0056	8.90	<0.01	1.05 (1.04−1.06)

VPD: Vapour pressure deficit: Aikake Information Criterion=1489.

of diagnostic plots similar to those shown in Fig. 7.1 (plots not shown). Deviance residuals were used to evaluate the Poisson model in this way since they should be approximately normally distributed. The diagnostics provided evidence of extra-Poisson variation in the data (i.e. overdispersion) and lack of normality in the distribution of the deviance residuals, suggesting that the model should be re-parameterized. A discussion of the methods for addressing these violations is provided in Section 7.4.

7.2.3 Logistic regression

As the level of resolution of our analyses becomes greater, that is, as the focus changes from a national to a regional or district level, the spatial unit of interest typically shifts from areas to points. Instead of describing and explaining disease counts summarized by area, the objective here is to identify factors that influence the risk of disease being present or absent at specific locations (e.g. farm or household) using the binary labels 'positive' (i.e. disease present) or 'negative' (i.e. disease absent).

When modelling binary data, explanatory variables are used to predict the probability of a study subject being disease positive (i.e. a 'case'). To do this, logistic regression models are used where the logit transform of the probability of the outcome (p) is modelled as a linear function of a set of explanatory variables (Breslow and Day 1987):

$$\log\left[\frac{p}{1-p}\right] = \beta_0 + \beta_1 x_{1i} + \ldots + \beta_m x_{mi} \quad (7.8)$$

Expressing the relationship between exposure and outcome in this way means that while the logit of

p might become very large or very small, the value of p can never extend beyond the bounds of zero and one. This transformation leads to the logistic model in which p can be expressed as a function of the m explanatory variables:

$$p = \frac{1}{1+e^{-(\beta_0 + \beta_1 x_{1i} + \ldots + \beta_m x_{mi})}} \quad (7.9)$$

To illustrate this method a subset of the British cattle TB data was used; specifically a region in the southwest of England where the prevalence of TB-positive farms is relatively high (Fig. 7.2). The 75 TB-positive holdings in this area were selected as cases and 225 control holdings were selected randomly from the 1,443 TB-negative holdings located within the boundaries of the study area. The location of case and control holdings is shown in Fig. 7.4.

In a study where the detection of spatial pattern is not of interest, cases and controls would be matched on the basis of known risk factors such as holding size, holding type, and location (Schlesselman 1982). However, if the detection of spatial pattern is of interest, matching controls by location is not useful since it would result in the spatial distribution of cases being the same (or similar) to that of the controls. A better approach, when the spatial distribution of disease is of interest, is to select controls so their spatial distribution closely matches the distribution of the underlying population at risk (Diggle 2003). Where individual units of interest are grouped by area (e.g. state or county) one would: (1) establish the number of controls required (based on sample size calculations to achieve a specified level of study power); (2) determine the number of controls required from each area in proportion to

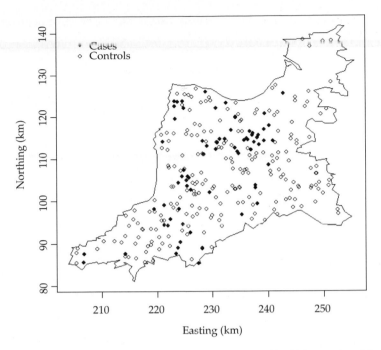

Figure 7.4 Point map showing the location of 75 TB-positive (•) and 225 TB-negative holdings (□) in a region of the southwest of England.

the total number of study units in each area; and (3) select the required number of units from each area using spatially random sampling. The success of this technique depends on the distribution of units within each area being uniformly distributed. As a rule of thumb, the areas chosen should be as small as possible because the smaller the area the greater the likelihood that units will be distributed uniformly within each area.

In this analysis the outcome of interest was the TB status of a holding (positive or negative) and once again, for parsimony, the analysis was restricted to explanatory variables related to atmospheric dryness and environmental temperature. Relationships between the outcome variable and each of the explanatory variables were visualized using box-and-whisker plots and quantified using the Kruskal–Wallis test. Variables were selected using the backward-stepwise approach and the final model is shown in Table 7.3.

Table 7.3 shows that the probability of a herd being TB-positive in this area is positively associated with the tri-annual amplitude and phase of the VPD, the VPD range, the amplitude of the annual

air temperature, and minimum air temperature, but negatively associated with mean VPD and the phase of the tri-annual air temperature. It should be noted that the explanatory variables and the magnitude of their effect on the odds of a holding being TB-positive differ from those estimated in the Poisson regression model (shown in Table 7.2). This could either be the result of ecological bias, as aggregating data at the area level fails adequately to represent the exposure response relationship for individual holdings within each area, or it could reflect epidemiological differences in the relationships between TB risk and the explanatory variables in this sub-area compared to the overall relationships for Great Britain. This model will be used again in Section 7.3.

7.2.4 Multilevel models

As already discussed, one of the key assumptions of linear, Poisson, and logistic regression is that of independence. The value of any response should be unrelated to any other response in the dataset. While this assumption may be valid for

Table 7.3 Point estimates and standard errors of regression coefficients in a fixed-effects logistic regression model of climatic factors influencing the presence of TB among holdings in a region of the southwest of England

Explanatory variable	Coefficient	SE	t	P-value	OR (95% CI)
Intercept	−130.7	45.43	−2.88	<0.01	
VPD mean	−0.1034	0.0314	−3.29	<0.01	0.90 (0.85–0.96)
VPD amplitude (tri-annual)	0.0802	0.0399	2.01	0.04	1.08 (1.00–1.18)
VPD phase (tri-annual)	0.2871	0.1215	2.36	0.02	1.33 (1.05–1.69)
VPD range	0.0294	0.0103	2.85	<0.01	1.03 (1.01–1.05)
Temperature amplitude (annual)	0.0929	0.0322	2.89	<0.01	1.10 (1.03–1.17)
Temperature minimum	0.0485	0.0155	3.13	<0.01	1.05 (1.02–1.08)
Temperature phase (tri-annual)	−0.0119	0.0035	−3.37	<0.01	0.99 (0.98–0.99)

VPD: Vapour pressure deficit: Aikake Information Criterion=297.

many situations in epidemiological research there are situations where the inherent structure in the responses measured renders the assumption of independence invalid. For example, to identify risk factors for lameness in dairy cattle a researcher might conduct a prospective cohort study of cows in 25 dairy herds. Cow-level details are collected including breed, age, date of calving, and date and details of each lameness event (if these occur). At the end of the study the researcher finds that the incidence of lameness varies widely among the 25 herds, which leads to the question: is the risk of lameness due to factors operating at the individual cow level (such as age, breed, or foot conformation) or the herd level (such as condition of farm raceways or the level of patience exercised by the herd manager)?

The most likely answer to this question is that the risk of lameness is due to a combination of both cow- and herd-level factors. Working out the contribution of each of these sources of variation on lameness risk is useful when attempting to control disease. If most of the variation in disease risk is due to individual (cow) level factors, then addressing individual-level exposures (e.g. age, breed, stage of lactation, and condition of feet) should be the most effective way to manage the problem. If on the other hand group-level (i.e. herd) factors account for most of the variation in disease risk, then attention to group-level exposures (e.g. condition of farm raceways) should provide a more effective disease management strategy.

To identify the relative contribution of individual and group-level factors on the overall risk of lameness, regression techniques must be adapted to account for the multilevel nature of the data. The term 'multilevel' in this context refers to the nested (or clustered) structure of the data. In this example, study subjects (cows) are clustered within herds. The implication here is that cows from the same herd have characteristics in common and are therefore not independent. Examples of multilevel data are found in the fields of education, medicine, and public health. Students are clustered within schools, patients are clustered within hospitals, individuals clustered within families, and households clustered within geographical regions. Although these are all examples of single hierarchies, multiple hierarchies are also possible (and common). For example, cows can be clustered within herds, herds clustered within farms, and farms clustered within regions. Depending on the underlying biological mechanism, subjects from within a cluster may be more alike than subjects from different clusters due to their shared environment. In a clustered dataset, observed values (e.g. measures of disease outcome) from within the same cluster are not independent. If this lack of independence is not accounted for, the population variance will be underestimated and it may be falsely concluded that a statistical association is present when in fact it is absent. To learn more about multilevel modelling the reader is referred to Goldstein (1995), Kreft and de Leeuw (1998), Snijders and Bosker (1999),

Leyland and Goldstein (2001), Browne (2005), or Gelman and Hill (2006).

What does all of this have to do with spatial epidemiology? Tobler's First Law of Geography states that 'Everything is related to everything else but near things are more related than distant things'. As discussed in Chapter 2, subjects that are close in space are likely to be similar and spatial proximity therefore represents a form of clustering (in the same way that cows are clustered within a herd and students are clustered within schools).

For outcomes measured on a continuous scale, the simplest multilevel model is a variance-components model. This is a variation of linear regression with the key difference being that the variable defining the cluster is treated as a random effect. Consider a study which monitors Y_{ij}, responses from i individuals that reside within j clusters (that is, there are i level 1 units and j level-2 units). These data can be expressed as a random intercepts model where Y_{ij} is the sum of a random intercept for the level-2 units j, β_{0j}, and the residual effect for the level-1 units within the level-2 units, ε_{ij}:

$$Y_{ij} = \beta_{0j} + \varepsilon_{ij} \qquad (7.10)$$

Assuming the ε_{ij} have a mean of zero, the term β_{0j} can be thought of as the mean of each of the level-2 units. Groups where β_{0j} is high tend to have (on average) high values of Y_{ij} and groups where β_{0j} is low tend to have (on average) low values of Y_{ij}. The level-2 component of (7.10) can be broken down into two components:

$$\beta_{0j} = \lambda_{00} + U_{0j} \qquad (7.11)$$

where β_{0j} depends on γ_{00} (the level-2 intercept) and U_{0j} (the level-2 error term which has a mean of zero). In (7.11) γ_{00} represents the grand mean for the population (the mean of the intercepts) and U_{0j} is the error term for level-2 (the deviation of each group mean from the grand mean), which has a mean of zero. When U_{0j} is large the conclusion is that there are large differences in Y_{ij} between groups. Combining (7.10) and (7.11) results in:

$$Y_{ij} = \lambda_{00} + U_{0j} + \varepsilon_{ij} \qquad (7.12)$$

and it is assumed that the level-2 (group) effects have a mean of zero and variance σ_{u0}^2, the level-1 effects have a mean of zero and variance σ_{ε}^2, and

the random variables U_{0j} and ε_{ij} are mutually independent

$$U_{0j} \sim N(0, \sigma_{u0}^2)$$
$$\varepsilon_{ij} \sim N(0, \sigma_{\varepsilon}^2) \qquad (7.13)$$

Another type of multilevel model is a *random slopes* model in which regression coefficients for each of the m explanatory variables are estimated for each level 2-unit. This allows the influence of each covariate to vary for each level-2 unit. Models with random slopes and random intercepts are possible. For further details see Browne (2005).

An example will help to explain these ideas further. An observational study was conducted to identify risk factors for TB in British cattle. Thirty-two holdings provided data for this study. In the logistic regression model, holding was included as a random effect similar to, but not exactly the same as, the parameterization shown in (7.10) and (7.13). The holding-level random effect terms were sorted in ascending order and plotted (along with their 95% confidence intervals), as shown in Fig. 7.5.

It is evident from Fig. 7.5 that the holding-level random effect terms are centred around a log odds of zero, which is expected, given that the distribution of the random-effect terms was specified as having a mean of zero (7.13). Of greater interest (in terms of providing insight into potential options for controlling TB in this population) is the variability of the random-effect terms. The random-effect terms in Fig. 7.5 are relatively small for some holdings (e.g. holdings 84, 14, and 24) whereas in others they are relatively large (e.g. 23, 53, and 72). This implies that there are (unmeasured) holding-level effects operating in holdings 84, 14, and 24 that reduce the individual cow-level risk of TB. Similarly, there are unmeasured, holding-level effects increasing the risk of TB for cattle in holdings 23, 53, and 72. Although it has been established that holding-level effects are present and that they vary among herds, their exact nature cannot be determined from the data. For example, important holding-level effects for TB might include the cattle purchasing behaviour of the herd manager or the proximity of the farm to vectors of TB. A rational approach in this situation would be to compare management practices in holdings identified as 'high' and 'low' risk

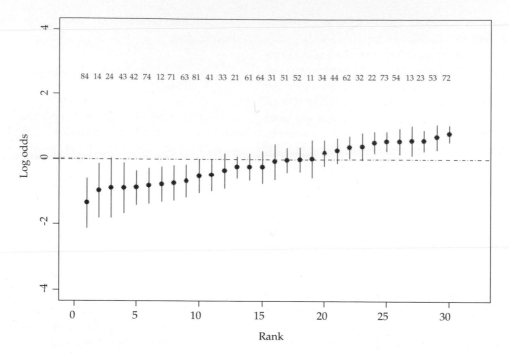

Figure 7.5 Caterpillar plot showing the point estimates and 95% confidence intervals of the holding-level random effect terms from a logistic regression model of individual cow and holding-level risks for TB in Great Britain. The numbers listed above each data point are the identifiers for each holding that took part in the study.

in order to identify more precisely the exact nature of the differences between the two groups.

A basic measure of the degree of dependency in multilevel data is the intraclass correlation coefficient (ICC, ρ). To continue with the model shown in (7.12), the total variance of Y_{ij} in the data is equal to the sum of the level-2 and level-1 variances:

$$\mathrm{var}(Y_{ij}) = \sigma_{u0}^2 + \sigma_\varepsilon^2 \qquad (7.14)$$

The covariance between the responses of two level-1 units in the same level-2 unit j is equal to the variance of the contribution U_{0j} shared by these level-2 units:

$$\mathrm{cov}(Y_{ij}, Y_{ji}) = \sigma_{u0}^2 \qquad (7.15)$$

and the correlation between values of two randomly drawn level-1 units in the same, randomly drawn level-2 unit is the ICC:

$$\mathrm{ICC} = \rho(Y_{ij}, Y_{i'j}) = \frac{\sigma_{u0}^2}{\sigma_{u0}^2 + \sigma_\varepsilon^2} \qquad (7.16)$$

The ICC provides a measure of the proportion of the variance in the outcome between the level-2 units. In a study where students (the level-1 units) are grouped within schools (the level-2 units), an ICC of 0.15 would mean that 15% of the variation in the outcome measure was due to differences between schools and 85% of the variation was due to differences between students.

Spatial proximity should be regarded as a form of clustering. When modelling spatial data a similar approach is adopted to that described in this section, the key difference being that the covariance matrix of the random-effect term is replaced with one incorporating the spatial structure of the data.

7.3 Accounting for spatial effects

In Chapter 2 the concepts of first-order (trend) and second-order (local) spatial effects were introduced as terms for describing the spatial characteristics of data. The term 'first-order' is used to describe large-scale variations in the mean of the outcome of interest due to location or other explanatory variables, while 'second-order' describes small-scale variation due to interactions between neighbours. The regression methods described here (linear, Poisson, and logistic) provide a means of quantifying first-order effects. Once the first-order effects have been accounted for, second-order effects can be investigated.

To identify the presence of unaccounted-for second-order effects, the residuals from each of the regression models developed should be examined for evidence of spatial autocorrelation using the methods described in Chapter 4. If there is no evidence of autocorrelation in the residuals then there is little point in trying to account for spatial dependency. In this case a model that does not account for spatial dependency should provide a satisfactory description of the data. If a second-order spatial pattern is evident in the residuals, the model can be extended to account for it. In this instance, a multilevel model is applied to the data treating spatial proximity as a form of clustering.

To illustrate this approach the residuals from the fixed effects Poisson model described in Section 7.2.2 were evaluated. As a first step, and informal check, the residual terms were plotted as a choropleth map (Fig. 7.6). This map showed aggregation of positive-sign residuals in the west of the Midlands and parts of the southwest of England. Confirmation of the presence of spatial autocorrelation in the residuals was provided by the Moran's I statistic ($I = 0.55$; $p < 0.01$). Recall from Chapter 4 that two items of data are required to calculate the Moran's I statistic: (1) a vector quantifying the outcome of interest for each area (in this case the area-level residuals), and (2) a spatial contiguity matrix defining each area's neighbours. In this example, the contiguity matrix was based on adjacency (i.e. neighbours were defined as areas sharing a common border). It was concluded, from the Moran's I statistic and Fig. 7.6, that the residuals from the Poisson regression model were spatially autocorrelated, indicating a lack of independence in the data (a violation of one of the assumptions of regression modelling) and that the model should be re-parameterized.

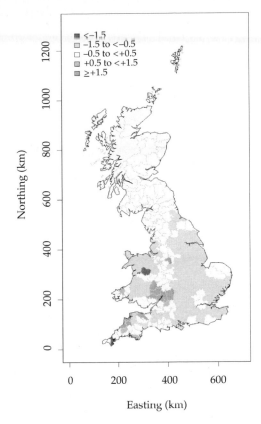

Figure 7.6 Choropleth map showing the spatial distribution of the area-level standardized residuals from the fixed-effects Poisson model of area-level TB risk in Great Britain shown in Table 7.2 See plate 9.

When dealing with point data, a variogram computed from the residuals is a useful way of identifying the presence of residual spatial autocorrelation. Fig. 7.7 shows a binned, omnidirectional variogram using the standardized residuals from the fixed-effects logistic regression model shown in Table 7.3. The dashed lines show the pointwise 95% limits constructed from 999 simulations where the residuals were randomly allocated to the case and control holding locations, and the empirical variogram computed for each simulation. The variogram for the observed data lies within the 95% limits throughout the plotted region, providing no evidence of unaccounted-for second-order structure in the data. This finding in itself provides important information in terms of understanding the between-holding transmission dynamics of TB

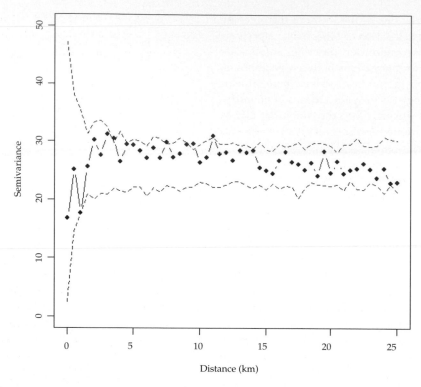

Figure 7.7 Binned omnidirectional variogram computed using the standardized residuals derived from the fixed-effects logistic regression model of TB risk shown in Table 7.3. The dashed lines show the pointwise 95% limits constructed from 999 simulations where the residuals were randomly allocated to the case and control holding locations, and the empirical variogram computed for each simulation.

in this area of Great Britain. After adjusting for the effect of various measures of atmospheric dryness and environmental temperature, there was no evidence of small-scale spatial pattern in the unexplained component of disease risk around any arbitrarily selected holding. This implies that (for this subset of the data at least) the risk of a herd being TB-positive is more dependent on herd-level characteristics (e.g. aspects of herd management), than on proximity to other TB-positive holdings. Given the absence of second-order effects, it may be that additional explanatory variables are required to account for the localized spatial pattern (that is, aggregation of TB-positive holdings in a particular area of the study region). Kernel smoothed intensity plots of the residuals from the fixed-effects model provide a starting point for investigating these influences further.

7.4 Area data

Typically there are two goals in modelling area data. Firstly, to quantify the influence of fixed effects on the level of disease within each area of a region under study and secondly, to identify areas where there are higher than expected counts of disease after the influence of specified fixed-effects have been accounted for. A number of techniques have been described to achieve these goals, ranging from frequentist approaches, which provide a global summary of the strength of area-to-area effect (see for example Walter et al. 1999), to full Bayesian mixed-effects models where area-level spatially correlated random effects are determined (see for example Toledano et al. 2001; Jarup et al. 2002).

This section focuses briefly on frequentist approaches to modelling area data and provides a more detailed description of the Bayesian methods that have been widely applied to spatial epidemiological problems in recent years (Lawson et al. 1999a).

7.4.1 Frequentist approaches

The first part of this chapter outlined the concepts behind linear, Poisson, and logistic regression modelling. These techniques represent the first phase of a spatial model-building exercise, allowing variables that explain all or part of the broad-scale (first-order) change in the mean of the outcome under investigation to be identified. As outlined in Section 7.3, the next step is to examine the fitted model for evidence of spatial autocorrelation in the residuals and, if present, to extend the model to account for this spatial dependency. In this instance, the linear regression model defined in 7.1 can be extended as follows:

$$\mu_i = \beta_0 + \beta_1 x_{1i} + \dots + \beta_m x_{mi} + \delta + \varepsilon_i \qquad (7.17)$$

where, μ_i is the outcome variable measured at location i, $\beta_0 + \beta_{1i} X_{1i} + \dots + \beta_{mi} X_{mi}$ represent the mean of the outcome variable at location i, and δ is a normally distributed random effect term with mean of zero and covariance matrix Σ, $\delta \sim N(0, \Sigma)$.

In a frequentist setting, three types of spatial covariance structures can be used to define Σ: conditional autoregressive (CAR), simultaneous autoregressive (SAR), and moving average (MA) models. In time-series analyses, autoregressive models are developed where observations are explained in terms of other observations that occurred in the recent past. For spatial data, a similar approach is used where observations are explained in terms of other, nearby observations. The covariance structures for CAR, SAR, and MA models are as follows:

$$\text{CAR:} \quad \Sigma = \frac{D\sigma^2}{(I - \rho W)} \qquad (7.18)$$

$$\text{SAR:} \quad \Sigma = \frac{\sigma^2}{(I - \rho W)^T D^{-1}(I - \rho W)} \qquad (7.19)$$

$$\text{MA:} \quad \Sigma = (I + \rho W)\, D(I + \rho W)^T \sigma^2 \qquad (7.20)$$

In (7.19), (7.20), and (7.21) ρ and σ are scalar parameters (estimated from the data), W is a weighted contiguity matrix, and D is a diagonal matrix used to account for non-constant variance of the marginal distributions. For each approach the spatial autocorrelation coefficient ρ provides a single measure of the strength of the interaction between neighbours after accounting for the explanatory variables included in the model. When the spatial contiguity matrix has been standardized to have row sums of unity, ρ will range from -1 to $+1$.

In Section 7.2.1 the relationship between median herd size in 178 areas of Great Britain and a set of environmental variables was explored (Table 7.1). Moran's I, computed for the residuals from the linear regression model shown in Table 7.1, provided evidence of spatial autocorrelation (results not shown). Table 7.4 shows the results from the same model with the key difference being that a CAR approach has been used to account for spatial autocorrelation in the data. Use of Moran's I statistic on the residuals from a linear model may, in some circumstances, not be valid. For further details the

Table 7.4 Point estimates and standard errors of the regression coefficients in a multiple conditional autoregressive (CAR) regression model of climatic factors influencing the median size of British cattle herds

Explanatory variable	Coefficient	SE	t	P-value
Intercept	−1,061.0	158.4	−6.69	<0.01
Elevation	−0.0696	0.0329	−2.11	0.03
Channel 3 amplitude (bi-annual)	−0.8047	0.2930	−2.74	<0.01
NDVI maximum	0.6711	0.0933	7.19	<0.01
VPD amplitude (bi-annual)	0.1077	0.0669	1.61	0.11

NDVI: Normalized Difference Vegetation Index, VPD: Vapour pressure deficit.

reader is referred to Ripley (1981) and Waller and Gotway (2004).

From a comparison of the fixed-effects model (Table 7.1) and the CAR model (Table 7.4), it is apparent firstly, that the estimated regression coefficients are closer to zero in the CAR model than in the fixed-effects model and secondly, that the estimated standard errors for all explanatory variables are larger in the CAR model. This is because in the CAR model, part of the variation in the data is explained by the spatial component of the model. The global spatial autocorrelation coefficient estimated for these data ($\rho = 0.166$) is indicative of weak to moderate correlation in herd size in areas defined as adjacent.

Residuals from the CAR model (as well as those from SAR and MA models) should follow a distribution that is approximately independently normal and should have constant variance. The diagnostic plot series described in Section 7.2.1 was applied to these data and confirmed this to be the case (results not shown). Moran's I statistic, computed using the residuals from the CAR model, provided a check to ensure that all spatial dependency in the data had been accounted for. In this instance, the null hypothesis of no spatial autocorrelation at the alpha level of 0.05 ($I = -0.08$; $P = 0.08$) was accepted.

Examples of the use of CAR and SAR models in the epidemiological literature include studies of regional variations in cancer incidence in Ontario, Canada (Walter et al. 1999), the relationship between exposure to air pollution and socioeconomic status in Hamilton, Ontario (Jerrett et al. 2001) and early childhood mortality in São Paulo, Brazil (Antunes and Waldman 2002). In their study, which investigated regional variations in cancer incidence, Walter et al. (1999) conclude that there is little change in the estimated risk coefficients after accounting for spatial autocorrelation, and that there are no areas of the province with systematically different cancer risks once known risk factors have been accounted for. In contrast, Jerrett et al. (2001), using a SAR approach, found that the significance of socio-economic indicators as predictors of particulate air pollution in Hamilton varied according to whether or not the model was adjusted to account for spatial autocorrelation. Jerrett et al.

(2001) conclude that it is important to account for spatial autocorrelation in health studies.

7.4.2 Bayesian approaches

A considerable literature has developed around Bayesian approaches to modelling disease counts at the small-area level (Manton et al. 1981; Tsutakawa 1988; Besag et al. 1991; Marshall 1991b; Clayton and Benardinelli 1992; Breslow and Clayton 1993; Lawson 1994; Ghosh et al. 1998). Central to this method is the inclusion of random-effect terms to account for unobserved, spatial features within the data. The appeal of this approach is that rather than producing a single (global) spatial autocorrelation coefficient (as in the case of the CAR, SAR, or MA approaches described in Section 7.4.1), spatially correlated random-effect terms are estimated for each area unit, thereby allowing the analyst to identify aggregations of spatial units where the incidence (or prevalence) of disease is not explained by the model.

For an overview of Bayesian methods in an epidemiological context, the reader is referred to either Spiegelhalter et al. (2002), or Lawson et al. (2003). Spiegelhalter et al. (2002) describes the Bayesian approach with particular reference to the analysis of clinical trial data. Lawson et al. (2003) describe Bayesian methods for disease mapping. For discussions of the methodological issues related to spatial epidemiology the reader is referred to Clayton and Kaldor (1987), Besag et al. (1991), Clayton and Benardinelli (1992), Cressie (1992), Devine et al. (1994a; 1994b), Pickle et al. (1996), Waller et al. (1997), Xia et al. (1997), Conlon and Louis (1999), Elliott et al. (2000), Banerjee et al. (2004), Gotway (2004), Waller and Gotway (2004), and Lawson (2006a).

Multilevel Bayesian models have been used to investigate the spatial distribution of testicular and prostate cancer in Britain (Toledano et al. 2001; Jarup et al. 2002), breast cancer in Greece (Vlachonikolis et al. 2002), insulin-dependent diabetes mellitus in Austria (Schober et al. 2001), stroke and cardiovascular disease in Great Britain (Maheswaran et al. 2002), multiple sclerosis in Italy (Pugliatti et al. 2002), low birth weights in Papua New Guinea (Müller et al. 2002), malaria in South

Africa (Kleinschmidt et al. 2002), and BSE in Great Britain (Stevenson et al. 2005).

In the discussion of models for Poisson-distributed outcomes in Section 7.2.2 it was explained that the mean number of disease events in spatial unit i can be explained in terms of m area-level covariates (7.6). In a Bayesian context, non-informative prior distributions can be assumed for the intercept β_0 and each of the m regression coefficients ($\beta_1, ..., \beta_m$). The exponent of β_i represents the residual relative risk in area i after adjusting for the m covariates included in the model. ε_i is interpreted as reflecting the residual variability between areas due to unknown or unmeasured risk factors. Unknown risk factors often vary in space, which in turn induces spatial correlation between the observed disease counts in each area and its neighbours. To account for this correlation it can be assumed that the unexplained variation comprises two parts; (1) a structured (spatially correlated); and (2) an unstructured (spatially random) component. An intermediate distribution of the log risk ratios, ranging from prior independence (unstructured heterogeneity) to prior local dependence (structured heterogeneity), is known as a convolution Gaussian prior (Besag 1989; Besag and Mollié 1989; Besag et al. 1991; Mollié 1996). In this context, the model may be parameterized as:

$$\log(\mu_i) = \log(n_i) + (\beta_0 + \beta_1 x_{1i} + ... + \beta_m x_{mi}) \\ + U_i + S_i + \xi_i \tag{7.21}$$

In (7.21), S_i represents the structured (spatially correlated) random effects and U_i represents the unstructured random effects for each of the i areas. It is usual to assume a spatially structured prior distribution for the structured component of the random effects. Various choices exist, but the most popular is a special case of the CAR model described by Besag et al. (1991). This models the log risk ratio in area i conditional on the risks in all other areas as being normally distributed about the weighted mean of the log risk ratio in the remaining areas, with the sum of the weights being inversely proportional to the variance σ^2. The unstructured heterogeneity component U_i is parameterized as being normally distributed with mean zero and variance τ^2. The strength of the 'mix' of structured and unstructured heterogeneity components depends

on the priors specified for σ^2 and τ^2. Large priors for σ^2 relative to τ^2 allow S_i to show wide variation (resulting in little spatial smoothing) whereas small priors for σ^2 relative to τ^2 forces all of the spatial heterogeneity terms to be similar (resulting in greater spatial smoothing). In practice, σ^2 and τ^2 are assigned prior distributions (hyperpriors) with a gamma distribution. Benardinelli et al. (1995), Best et al. (1999), and Richardson and Monfort (2000) discuss issues associated with the parameterization of hyperpriors in a spatial modelling context, concluding that the sensitivity of proposed models should be tested against a range of hyperprior specifications.

The study by Stevenson et al. (2005) illustrates the Bayesian hierarchical approach to modelling spatial data and provides an example of the additional insights that can be achieved by accounting for (and describing) spatial dependence in a dataset. These authors investigate factors influencing the distribution of BSE cases in Great Britain for cattle born either before or after the introduction of the July 1988 ban on feeding meat and bone meal to ruminants. Models are developed to quantify the effect of the following variables on the number of BSE-affected cattle in each of 178 areas of Great Britain during the two phases of the epidemic: (1) the ratio of dairy to non-dairy cattle; (2) the ratio of pigs to cattle; and (3) the northing of an area's centroid. Pig-to-cattle ratio is used as a covariate in an attempt to account for the proportional increase in post-control BSE counts from the east of the country, the hypothesis being that high-protein concentrate feeds produced in areas with large numbers of pigs (predominantly in the east of England) contaminates cattle feed manufactured and distributed in those areas, resulting in higher risk ratios for BSE.

The model building approach adopted by these authors follows the approach outlined in this chapter. Firstly, fixed-effect models are developed and then, owing to the presence of significant spatial autocorrelation in the residual terms, Bayesian mixed-effects models accounting for the structured (spatially correlated) and unstructured heterogeneity in the data are developed. A series of spatial contiguity matrices are considered, including those based on contiguity and distance. To account for edge effects the ratio of the length of each area's coastline to its total perimeter was determined, and the weights specified from the contiguity matrix multiplied by one minus the coastline-to-perimeter ratio for each district pair (Lawson 2006a). Correcting for edge effects produced risk ratios that were closer to unity, compared with those where no correction was made. Correcting for edge-effects therefore provided a more conservative estimate of the magnitude of the risk ratios for each of the fixed effects.

Details of the final models are shown in Table 7.5 and box-and-whisker plots of the estimated risk ratios for both the fixed- and mixed-effects models are shown in Fig. 7.8.

Table 7.5 and Fig. 7.8 show that unit increases in area-level pig-to-cattle ratio did not influence BSE risk for the pre-control cohort (relative risk 1.01,

95% credible interval 1.00–1.02) and had a positive influence on BSE risk for the post-control cohort (relative risk 1.06, 95% credible interval 1.04–1.08), consistent with the stronger effect of cross-contamination as a determinant of disease after the July 1988 feed ban. Choropleth maps of area-level risk ratios attributable to the structured heterogeneity terms from the mixed-effects model identified areas in the east, north, and southeast of England where there were (unmeasured) spatial aggregations of BSE risk not explained by dairy-to-non-dairy ratio, pig-to-cattle ratio, or area northing (Fig. 7.9b). Stevenson et al. (2005) speculate that the distribution of the unmeasured, spatially aggregated influences are consistent with the distribution of feed mills and/or compounders who failed fully to comply with the directives of the legislated control measures. The strength of this analytical approach

Table 7.5 Posterior means and standard deviations of the regression coefficients in the mixed-effects models of factors influencing area-level relative risk of bovine spongiform encephalopathy (BSE). Reproduced from Stevenson et al. (2005), with permission from *Preventive Veterinary Medicine*

Explanatory variable	Posterior mean	SD	MC error[a]	RR (95% CI)
Pre-control cohort[b]				
Intercept	0.5224	0.2888	0.03	
Ratio dairy: non-dairy	0.0239	0.0055	< 0.01	1.02 (1.01–1.04)
Ratio pigs: cattle	0.0102	0.0073	< 0.01	1.01 (1.00–1.02)
Northing[c]	−0.2518	0.0754	0.01	0.78 (0.67–0.89)[d]
Heterogeneity				
Structured[e]	0.4133	0.0777	0.01	
Unstructured[e]	0.1546	0.0607	< 0.01	
Post-control cohort[f]				
Intercept	0.8138	0.1027	< 0.01	
Ratio dairy: non-dairy	0.0255	0.0106	< 0.01	1.03 (1.00–1.05)
Ratio pigs: cattle	0.0571	0.0083	< 0.01	1.06 (1.04–1.08)
Northing	−0.3756	0.0366	< 0.01	0.69 (0.66–0.72)
Heterogeneity				
Structured[e]	0.3653	0.0366	< 0.01	
Unstructured[e]	0.4467	0.0132	< 0.01	

[a] Monte Carlo error.

[b] Structured heterogeneity terms based on a spatial contiguity matrix where areas are defined as neighbours if they share a common border.

[c] 100 km increments.

[d] Interpretation: for 100 km increases in the northing coordinate of an area's centroid, area-level risk of BSE was reduced by a factor of 0.74 (95% credible interval 0.61–0.89).

[e] Variance of heterogeneity term.

[f] Structured heterogeneity terms based on a spatial contiguity matrix where areas are defined as neighbours if the Euclidean distance between area centroids was less than 100 km.

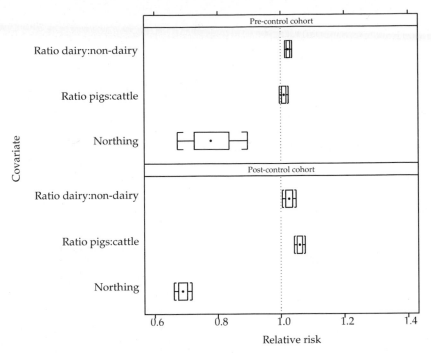

Figure 7.8 Box-and-whisker plots showing the 95% credible interval of the relative risk estimates for the fixed-effect and mixed-effects model of area-level bovine spongiform encephalopathy (BSE) risk for the pre- and post-control cohorts. Adapted from Stevenson et al. (2005), with permission from *Preventive Veterinary Medicine*.

is that it allows one to distinguish between factors fixed in their influence on BSE risk from area to area (i.e. dairy-to-non-dairy ratio, pig-to-cattle ratio, and northing) and unmeasured factors that varied spatially. Mapping these unmeasured factors indicates where the presence of disease was unaccounted for, telling authorities where to look for previously unrecognized BSE risks. Of particular note is that these areas (as shown in Fig. 7.9b) were not in those areas of the country where the SMR for BSE was highest (Fig. 7.9a).

Mixture models, as described by Böhning and Schlattmann (1992) and Schlattmann (1996a; 1996b), are a variation of the Bayesian hierarchical models described in this chapter and assume that areas within a study region can be grouped into discrete homogeneous risk classes. These models force those areas within a group to have the same structured heterogeneity terms, imposing a discontinuity in spatially-structured risk between one group and the next. While these models address

the issue of discontinuities that may legitimately exist in some situations, for example, at urban–rural fringes, they do not account for the possibility that areas within a study region may also have smooth rate transitions. Developing this concept, Lawson and Clark (2002) describe a special type of spatial mixture model that allows for different forms of spatial variation, linked by a spatially varying weights matrix. Models of this type provide a flexible compromise between the fixed spatial weighting scheme used by Besag et al. (1991) and the homogeneous risk class scheme used by Böhning and Schlattmann (1992), Schlattmann (1996a; 1996b).

7.5 Point data

7.5.1 Frequentist approaches

Models of spatial point data seek to quantify the influence of a set of explanatory variables on the

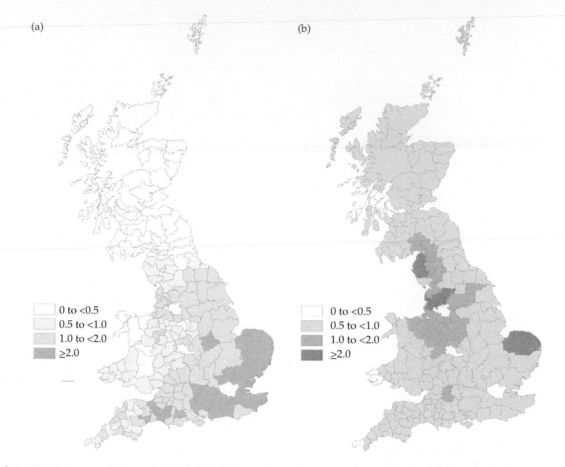

Figure 7.9 Bovine spongiform encephalopathy (BSE) in the population of cattle present in Great Britain from 30 June 1986 to 30 June 1997. Choropleth maps showing: (a) area-level standardized mortality ratios (SMRs) for BSE in the post-control cohort (cattle born between 18 July 1988 and 30 June 1997), and (b) the exponential structured heterogeneity terms from the mixed-effects model for the post-control cohort. Reproduced from Stevenson et al. (2005), with permission from *Preventive Veterinary Medicine*.

occurrence of events throughout a study region, taking into account spatial dependency. Typically these techniques have been applied to putative sources of hazard where the number of disease events in a region of study are enumerated for a defined period and the spatial distribution of cases in relation to a hypothesised hazard is assessed (see for example Diggle and Rowlingson 1994; Lawson and Williams 1994; Diggle and Elliott 1995; Viel et al. 1995, Lawson and Clark 1999).

Heterogeneous Poisson Process (HEPP) techniques provide a way of modelling the spatial distribution of point events (Lawson 1989; Baddeley and Turner 2000; Diggle 2003). HEPP models are based on three assumptions. Firstly, individuals within a specified study population behave independently with respect to disease propensity, secondly, that the population at risk from which cases arise has a continuous spatial distribution, and thirdly, case events are unique in that they occur as single, spatially separate events. Within this framework the density of case events at any point can be parameterized as:

$$\lambda(y) = \varsigma \cdot g(y) \cdot f(y;\varphi) \qquad (7.22)$$

In (7.22) ς represents the risk of disease across the entire study area, $g(y)$ is a function representing the spatial distribution of the population throughout the study area, and $f(y;\varphi)$ is a relative risk function (which may include explanatory variables quantifying the effect of factors influencing the probability of disease at a given location, such as proximity to a hypothesized pollution source). A variety of relationships may be defined for the relative risk function $f(y;\varphi)$. Firstly, risk might vary with distance r from a specified source:

$$f(y;\varphi) = 1 + \exp^{-\beta r} \qquad (7.23)$$

Alternatively, it might be appropriate to parameterize risk in terms of direction from a hypothesized source as well as distance (Lawson and Williams 1994; Lawson 1995; Viel et al. 1995; Le et al. 1996):

$$f(y;\varphi) = 1 + \exp^{\beta_1 \log_e r - \beta_2 r + \cos\theta + \sin\theta} \qquad (7.24)$$

An attractive feature of the HEPP approach is that it can be used for focused clustering assessments, where a cluster centre is identified *a priori* and a model developed to determine the significance of this location as a cluster centre. In this situation, (7.22) can be re-parameterized as:

$$\lambda(y) = \varsigma \cdot g(y) \cdot m \left\{ \sum_{j=1}^{k} h_1(y - y_j) \right\} \qquad (7.25)$$

to describe the intensity of events around k centres located at y_j. Here the function $f(\cdot)$ is replaced by a link function m. The distribution of events around each hypothesized cluster centre is defined by the cluster distribution function $h_1(\cdot)$ which may be specified separately for each cluster. Lawson and Clark (1999) provide an example of this approach using infant lymphoma and leukaemia diagnoses in Humberside, England. In agreement with the findings of earlier analyses of the same data (Cuzick and Edwards 1990; Diggle and Chetwynd 1991), they find little support for a positive number of cluster centres.

HEPP models can be fitted within standard generalized linear model packages using special integration schemes (Berman and Turner 1992; Lawson 1992; Baddeley and Turner 2000). The spatstat package (Baddeley and Turner 2002) implemented in R (R Development Core Team 2006) provides functions for fitting HEPP models. Although primarily intended for ecological applications, this package offers a set of tools eminently suitable for applications in spatial epidemiology.

An alternative to HEPP techniques is provided by generalized additive models (Hastie and Tibshirani 1990). For binary responses a generalized additive model may be expressed as an additive logistic model:

$$\log\left[\frac{p}{1-p}\right] = \beta_0 + \beta_1 x_{1i} + \ldots + \beta_m x_{mi} + S(y_i) \qquad (7.26)$$

In (7.26) α represents the intercept, $\beta_1 x_{1i} + \ldots + \beta_m x_{mi}$ represent the regression coefficients for m explanatory variables and $S(y_i)$ provides a measure of the risk of disease at location y after accounting for the m explanatory variables. In a generalized additive model setting the only assumption about S is that it is a smooth function of y. Kelsall and Diggle (1998) use this approach to investigate the spatial distribution of cancer diagnoses in Walsall, an area in the north of England. They conclude that although the generalized additive model approach is computationally more demanding than other methods it has the advantage of allowing any number of explanatory variables to be controlled for. There are few examples of the generalized additive model methodology in the medical and veterinary spatial epidemiological literature. In contrast, the technique appears to be used relatively frequently in marine biology to quantify aspects of fish abundance (Borchers et al. 1997; Bellido et al. 2001; Zheng et al. 2002).

7.5.2 Bayesian approaches

Bayesian approaches may also be applied to the modelling of point data. Following on from the description provided in Section 7.4.2, each point in a region of study can be regarded as a set of individual 'areas' and, depending on the nature of the outcome variable measured at each point, any of the models discussed in Section 7.2 (linear, Poisson, or logistic) can be applied to the data. A contiguity matrix (based on distance) might then be used to account for second-order effects. While this is directly analogous to the approach used to model area data and is conceptually simple, a major drawback with it is that the contiguity matrix can become extremely large (and complex) as the number of point locations in the dataset increases.

An alternative is to develop logistic geostatistical models of the form:

$$\log\left[\frac{p}{1-p}\right] = \beta_0 + \beta_1 x_{1i} + \ldots + \beta_m x_{mi} + S(y_i) + \xi_i$$

(7.27)

where y_i represents the location of each point. In (7.27) the term $S(y_i)$ represents a structured (spatially correlated) heterogeneity term that is allowed to vary continuously through space (rather than discretely as in the case of models generally used for area data) and is based on a zero mean Gaussian process with variance σ^2. The geoR (Ribeiro Jr and Diggle 2001; Diggle and Ribeiro Jr 2007), and geoRglm (Christensen et al. 2002; Diggle and Ribeiro Jr 2007) packages implemented within R provide functionality for fitting Poisson log-linear and binary logistic geostatistical models, respectively.

Diggle et al. (2002) apply a binary logistic linear geostatistical model to a study of risk factors for childhood malaria in Gambia, in which the presence of malarial parasites in a blood sample is parameterized in terms of child-level covariates, village-level covariates, and separate components for residual spatial and non-spatial extra-binomial variation. Diggle et al. (2002) conclude that the dominant component of extra-binomial variation in these data is spatially structured, suggesting that the unexplained risk of malaria is due to environmental factors rather than non-spatial factors (such as familial susceptibility). Clements et al. (2006a) use a binary logistic geostatistical model as a tool for planning and implementing control programmes for schistosomiasis in Tanzania. The authors use remotely sensed data to identify and quantify factors associated with the presence of disease in school children. Differences in the spatially correlated component of infection risk for *Schistosoma haematobium* and *S. mansoni* are identified and the authors conclude that these differences are due to environmental requirements of the respective intermediate

hosts. In a further study, Clements et al. (2006b) use binary logistic geostatistical models to predict schistosomiasis infection intensity in East Africa, in contrast to the earlier study where the aim was to develop a model explaining disease risk. Additional examples of the application of geostatistical models applied to the epidemiology of schistosomiasis are provided by Raso et al. (2005), Raso et al. (2006a), and Yang et al. (2005). Raso et al. (2006b), in a study of risk factors for hookworm infection among school children in a rural area of western Côte d'Ivoire, assume non-stationarity in the underlying spatial dependence, allowing it to vary as a function of both distance and location.

7.6 Continuous data

7.6.1 Trend surface analysis

Trend surface analyses involve the application of a polynomial function of the spatial coordinates of sample sites to the observed data values using ordinary least squares or non-parametric regression. Covariates other than location may be included in the model to further understand or explain spatial variation. This technique is illustrated using the herd size data introduced in Section 7.2.1. As a first step the spatial structure of herd size was explored by looking at scatterplots of median herd size as a function of easting and northing coordinates of an area's centroid (Fig. 7.10), and adding non-parametric regression curves to identify trends in the data. These plots showed that median herd sizes are greatest in the west (areas with an easting coordinate between 200 and 400 km) and in the north (areas with a northing coordinate between 500 and 800 km) of Britain. An image plot of predicted herd size, computed using the easting and northing coordinates of each area's centroid as predictors in a non-parametric locally weighted (loess) regression model is shown in Fig. 7.11.

Fig. 7.11 provides a readily interpretable representation of the spatial distribution of median herd size throughout Great Britain, showing that larger herds (greater than 75 cattle) are located in the west of England, specifically in the counties of Somerset, Wiltshire, Dorset, and Cheshire, and in the south of Scotland. Although the loess model captures the

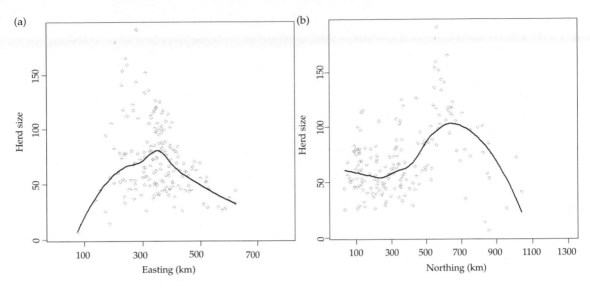

Figure 7.10 Scatterplots of median size of cattle herds in Great Britain as a function of the (a) easting coordinate of each area's centroid and (b) northing coordinate of each area's centroid.

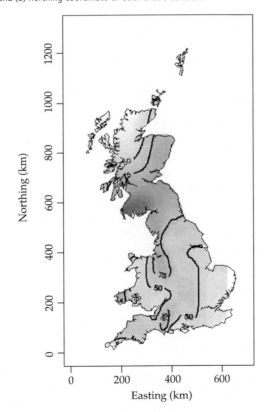

Figure 7.11 Image plot of predicted median herd size, computed using the easting and northing coordinates of each area's centroid as predictors in a non-parametric locally weighted (loess) regression model.

broad-scale spatial trend in herd size, it is reasonable to assume that herd size might be spatially autocorrelated at small spatial scales due to factors such as the price of land, proximity to markets and feed companies, and climate. This possibility was investigated by constructing an empirical, omni-directional variogram which provides evidence of spatial autocorrelation in median herd size up to a distance of around 80 km (Fig. 7.12a). To evaluate how well the loess model accounts for the second-order properties in the data, a variogram based on the model residuals was constructed. The variogram shown in Fig. 7.12b is essentially flat, providing evidence that the loess trend surface model accounts for most of the second-order spatial variation in the data.

Moore (1999) uses trend surface analyses to identify the direction and speed of diffusion of an epidemic of raccoon-rabies in Pennsylvania, USA between 1982 and 1986. Acknowledging the caveats involved in applying this technique to spatial data, Moore (1999) concludes that the technique is useful for removing the inherent noise in the reported data and helps to identify geographic 'corridors' within Pennsylvania that are associated with higher rates of diffusion of the disease. Hanchette and Schwartz (1992) use trend surface

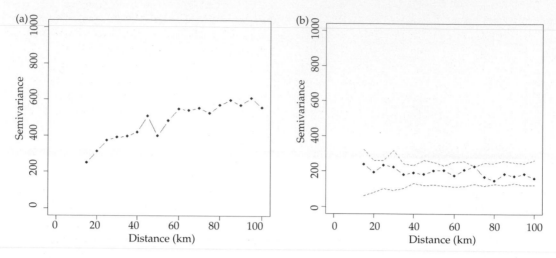

Figure 7.12 Omnidirectional variograms computed using (a) median herd size for each area and (b) the residuals derived from the loess model described in the text. The dashed lines in (b) show the pointwise 95% limits constructed from 999 simulations where the residuals were randomly allocated an area location and the variogram computed for each simulation.

analyses to assess geographic patterns in prostate cancer mortality in the United States, identifying a north–south trend thought to be consistent with the hypothesis that exposure to ultraviolet radiation is protective against the disease.

7.6.2 Generalized least squares models

An assumption of trend surface analyses is that model residuals are (spatially) independent. While this is the case in the herd size analysis presented in the previous section there are many occasions when this is not the case, particularly when dealing with environmental data such as rainfall or temperature. In this situation generalized least squares models provide the ability to account for lack of residual independence.

Given the general expression for a linear regression model shown in (7.1) it can be said (when modelling spatial data) that the $\beta_m x_{mi}$ terms represent the first-order component of the spatial process and ε_i represents a zero mean vector of errors with variance-covariance matrix C. Although ε_i has a mean of zero, the values of ε_i at different locations are not necessarily independent, having a covariance function defined by the term C. To produce an appropriate spatial generalized least squares regression model for continuous data the elements

of C need to be estimated directly. This is done by considering the variogram functions developed to explore the second-order properties of the data (as discussed in Chapter 6).

Three variogram models are commonly used for stationary spatial processes: (1) spherical; (2) exponential; and (3) Gaussian. In practice, a variogram is computed using the residuals from a fixed-effects model, and then some form of nonlinear least squares optimization is applied to derive a satisfactory model of the empirical variogram. For further details, and access to a comprehensive set of tools for applying these techniques, the reader is referred to the geoR package in R (Ribeiro Jr and Diggle 2001; Diggle and Ribeiro Jr 2007) or the SpatialStats module in S-Plus (Kaluzny et al. 1996).

Having developed a satisfactory variogram model for the error terms, a covariance matrix (based on the variogram model) can be included in the model parameterization. In effect this 'corrects' the parameter estimates and standard errors of the generalized least squares regression for second-order effects. This approach is applied (for illustrative purposes) to the herd size model. In Section 7.2.1 a linear regression model of factors influencing the median size of cattle herds in 178 areas throughout Great Britain was developed. Analysis of the residual terms from this model showed that their variance was not constant (Fig. 7.1a). Fig. 7.13 shows the empirical, omnidirectional variogram computed on the residual terms for the model presented in Table 7.1. Shown in Fig. 7.13 is an exponential model of the empirical variogram, computed using weighted least squares in the variofit function in the geoR package (Ribeiro Jr and Diggle 2001; Diggle and Ribeiro Jr 2007). A generalized least squares model was applied to the data using the exponential variogram model to account for spatial autocorrelation in the data. The final model is shown in Table 7.6.

It can be seen that the generalized least squares model (Table 7.6), which accounts for spatial autocorrelation, provides regression coefficients that are

closer to zero and have larger standard errors, than the multiple linear regression model (Table 7.1). This occurs as a result of part of the variation in the data being accounted for by the presence of spatial autocorrelation and means that the estimated effect of each of the explanatory variables on median herd size is not as large as in the first (simpler) analysis.

7.7 Discriminant analysis

In contrast to the regression methods discussed so far in this chapter, which seek a least-squares or error-minimizing description of epidemiological data, discriminant analysis seeks to maximize some between- to within-sample variance or other measure of spread around the sample means. In this case the 'samples' are not dealt with as continuous variables but as categorical ones. Presence or absence of disease is clearly categorical but other epidemiological variables, such as incidence or prevalence, can be turned into a series of categories (low, medium, and high) without too much loss of information. Indeed, some continuous epidemiological data such as malaria prevalence, are automatically turned into risk categories by clinicians who recognize only a small set of distinct clinical outcomes and treatment options. It then becomes important to choose category boundaries that make clinical rather than statistical sense. Sample sizes that are too small may render some discriminant techniques inapplicable.

Discriminant analysis assumes a multivariate normal distribution of the descriptor data around each categorical sample mean. Although other distributions are theoretically possible, there appear to

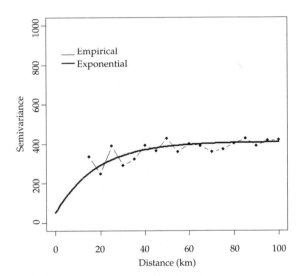

Figure 7.13 Omnidirectional variogram for the median cattle herd size data.

Table 7.6 Point estimates and standard errors of the regression coefficients of a generalized least squares model of climatic factors influencing the median size of British cattle herds

Explanatory variable	Coefficient	SE	t	P-value
Intercept	−598.1	163.0	−3.66	<0.01
Elevation	−0.0633	0.0583	−1.09	0.27
Channel 3 amplitude (bi-annual)	−0.0672	0.4162	−0.16	0.87
NDVI maximum	0.3926	0.0963	4.08	<0.01
VPD amplitude (bi-annual)	−0.0005	0.0829	−0.01	0.99

NDVI: Normalized Difference Vegetation Index.

be no applications of them in epidemiology. Many epidemiological data are clearly not multivariate normal but can be rendered more so by clustering the entire dataset on the basis of the descriptor variables. Most clustering algorithms emphasize between- to within-cluster differences and some even seek to maximize these differences. Thus, each of several clusters contributing to a dataset is more nearly multivariate normal than is the entire unclustered dataset. Formal tests for assessing the multivariate normality of the clusters exist (Bartlett 1947) but are rarely used. Although the following discussion focuses on the discrimination of the presence or absence of a disease, the same approach can be applied to categorical incidence or prevalence data.

Discriminant analysis usually involves three steps. Firstly, the covariance of the predictor variable values for a set of sample observations of known presence or absence status is calculated. This effectively defines the characteristics of the multivariate normal distribution around each centroid. Secondly, these covariances are used to test the accuracy of discrimination of the observations that were used to define the multivariate distributions. Ideally, the original observations are divided into two groups: a 'training set' used to define the multivariate distributions in the first step and an independent 'testing set' to test the accuracy of discrimination based on the distributions defined in the second step. In the final step new areas are classified as 'presence' or 'absence' sites on the basis of the values for them of the same predictor variables that were selected in the first two steps. It is assumed that the accuracy of the predictions made in this third step is equivalent to that of the testing set sample in the second step. This is not guaranteed however, since the training and testing set observations may have been collected in a different way or a different place from those of the new observations, and it is important to examine any indication of this.

In its simplest form, discriminant analysis assumes a common within-group covariance of the variables for all points defining both disease presence and absence. If $\bar{x}_{1v}$ is the (column vector) mean of a multivariate distribution involving v variables that define the absence of a disease, and $\bar{x}_{2v}$ is the

equivalent mean defining the presence of the disease, then the multivariate measure of separation between these two means is the Mahalanobis distance, D^2, defined as follows:

$$\begin{aligned} D^2{}_{12} &= (\bar{x}_1 - \bar{x}_2)' C_w^{-1} (\bar{x}_1 - \bar{x}_2) \\ &= d' C_w^{-1} d \end{aligned}$$

(7.28)

where $d = (\bar{x}_1 - \bar{x}_2)$, the apostrophe (') indicates the transpose and C_w^{-1} is the inverse of the within-groups covariance (dispersion) matrix C_w (Green 1978). Inspection of (7.28) shows that the Mahalanobis distance is no more than the squared Euclidean distance between two points in multivariate space $(ED^2{}_{12} = (\bar{x}_1 - \bar{x}_2)'(\bar{x}_1 - \bar{x}_2)$ adjusted for the covariance of variables (assumed to be the same) around each mean. Since probability is a non-linear but continuously declining function of increasing Mahalanobis distance it is possible to assign multivariate observations to the presence or absence category simply on the basis of their Mahalanobis distance values. Each observation is assigned to whichever category has the lower Mahalanobis distance value. However, it is usually helpful to make more probabilistic statements of presence and absence. The Mahalanobis distance may be used within the formula for a multivariate normal distribution to define the probability directly (D^2 is distributed as χ^2 with $(v-1)$ degrees of freedom where v, as before, is the number of variables defining each centroid). This probability involves all the remaining terms of the multivariate probability distribution formula, but since it is usually the probability with which any particular multivariate observation belongs to each of a defined set of outcomes (e.g. presence or absence) that is required, it is more usual to normalize each probability by dividing it by the sum of all probabilities, so that the sum of all predicted probabilities is one. This calculation produces what are called 'posterior probabilities', defined for two groups, $g = 1, 2$ (e.g. presence/absence), as follows:

$$P(1 \mid x) = \frac{p_1 e^{-D^2{}_1/2}}{\displaystyle\sum_{g=1}^{2} p_g e^{-D^2{}_g/2}}$$

and

$$P(2|x) = \frac{p_2 e^{-D^2_2/2}}{\sum\limits_{g=1}^{2} p_g e^{-D^2_g/2}} \qquad (7.29)$$

where $P(1|x)$ is the posterior probability that observation x belongs to group 1 and $P(2|x)$ the posterior probability that it belongs to group 2 (Green 1978) (the exponential terms in (7.29) are those of the multivariate normal distribution defining groups 1 and 2). All other terms of the multivariate distributions are the same in both the numerator and denominator and therefore cancel out (Tatsuoka 1971). In (7.29), p_1 and p_2 are the prior probabilities of belonging to the same two groups respectively. In the absence of any prior experience it is usual to assume equal prior probabilities of belonging to any of the groups and therefore, in the simple case of two-group discrimination, $p_1 = p_2 = 0.5$.

It should be emphasized that normalization in (7.29) will produce an allocation to one or other of the categories regardless of whether or not an allocation should be made. If for example, a new observation is a long way in multivariate space from any of the defined centroids, it will be allocated to one or other of them by the normalization step. It is best to avoid predictions in this case, and this may be done by deciding that observations with Mahalanobis distances greater than those seen in the training set should be assigned to a new category indicating that no prediction is possible for them.

In general, output predictions are required in the form of images called 'risk maps' (maps of the probability of environmental suitability for the vector or disease in question). It is advisable to produce, with this output image, a second image of the Mahalanobis distance to the nearest cluster in the training set (i.e. the cluster to which each pixel is assigned). This image can then be examined to find areas where the Mahalanobis distances are very large and where predictions are therefore likely to be inaccurate.

As indicated earlier, (7.28) and (7.29) should be modified when the assumption of common covariances is obviously invalid. Not only may areas of presence and absence differ in their environmental characteristics, but different parts of a species range may also show more subtle differences, requiring separate multivariate descriptions of their environmental conditions. Separate cluster analysis of the environmental variables defining presence and absence is performed here using the *k-means cluster* algorithm of the SPSS statistical package (SPSS Inc. Chicago, Illinois). Each cluster (either for presence or absence) is then treated as a separate multivariate normal distribution with its own covariance characteristics, and the posterior probabilities are calculated by summing across all distributions. In the case of two groups only (one for presence and one for absence), (7.29) is modified as follows:

$$P(1|x) = \frac{p_1 |C_1|^{-1/2} e^{-D^2_1/2}}{\sum\limits_{g=1}^{2} p_g |C_g|^{-1/2} e^{-D^2_g/2}}$$

and

$$P(2|x) = \frac{p_2 |C_2|^{-1/2} e^{-D^2_2/2}}{\sum\limits_{g=1}^{2} p_g |C_g|^{-1/2} e^{-D^2_g/2}} \qquad (7.30)$$

where $|C_1|$ and $|C_2|$ are the determinants of the covariance matrices for groups one and two respectively. The Mahalanobis distances in (7.30), calculated from (7.28), are evaluated using the separate within-group co-variance matrices C^1 and C^2 (Tatsuoka 1971). When there is more than a single class of presence or absence data (e.g. multiple clusters) the summation in the denominator of (7.30) covers the entire set of $g > 2$ groups and there are as many posterior probability equations as there are groups. With unequal covariance matrices the discriminant axis (strictly speaking a plane) that separates the two groups in multivariate space is no longer linear and (7.30) then effectively defines the maximum likelihood solution to the problem (Swain 1978). Inclusion of prior probabilities makes these predictions Bayesian.

Clustering is usually beneficial in the analyses described here and increases the fit of the discriminant analysis models, but it should never be allowed to produce clusters with less than a minimum number of data points since this results in badly defined covariance matrices (which sometimes cannot be inverted) and inaccurate predictions. A single faulty covariance matrix can affect all outputs of the discriminant analysis models.

In (7.30), the use of observed (generally training-set) prior probabilities shifts the equi-probability contours towards the smaller groups, resulting in a larger proportion of assignments to the classes with larger group sizes. This shift generally increases predictive accuracy. Further details of multivariate analysis may be found in several useful texts including Tatsuoka (1971), Green (1978), Krzanowski and Marriott (1995) and Legendre and Legendre (1998).

7.7.1 Variable selection within discriminant analysis

Whilst it is possible to use all available variables within discriminant analysis this is neither desirable nor efficient as biological interpretation of the importance of many contributory variables is very difficult, and statistical parsimony is lost. Predictor variables may be selected in numerous ways to maximize or minimize certain desirable statistical criteria. Since the process is one of discrimination, both the sensitivity and specificity of the results are of interest rather than either of these alone. Variables could therefore be selected on the basis of jointly maximizing these criteria, but often other metrics are used, commonest amongst which are the kappa index of agreement, the receiver-operating characteristic (ROC) curve, the area under the curve (AUC), or one of a number of different information criteria such as Akaike's (Rogers (2006) gives a table of these). Kappa is designed to measure predictive accuracy taking into account the correct predictions that would arise entirely by chance. Its value varies from –1 to +1 with a value of zero indicating a fit no better than random and a value of one indicating a perfect fit to the data. It has recently been shown that the kappa index of agreement is quite variable when percentage positives are either very low or very high and is most

reliable when there is the same number of positive and negative observations in the training set (McPherson et al. 2004). The AUC or ROC curve approach plots sensitivity against (1-specificity). It varies between zero and one with higher values indicating a better fit. Both kappa and AUC/ROC are calculated from the categorical predictions of the model but other accuracy statistics are based on its probabilistic predictions. The Kullback–Leibler (K–L) information or distance measure is a measure of the distance between a model and reality, and the smaller the distance the more the model captures that reality. Akaike (1973) showed that in practice the K–L distance could be estimated from the empirical log-likelihood function evaluated at its maximum point, to produce the Akaike Information Criterion (AIC) which is defined as follows:

$$AIC = -2 \log (\lambda(\hat{\theta}|y)) + 2K \qquad (7.31)$$

where $log(\ell(\theta|y))$ is the value of the log-likelihood at its maximum point (i.e. the maximum likelihood estimate) and K is the number of estimated parameters in the model. The first term on the right-hand side of (7.31) will tend to decrease as the number of parameters in the model increases (generally models with more parameters fit datasets better than those with fewer parameters), whilst the second term ($2K$) will obviously increase. This achieves a balance between over-fitting and under-fitting a model.

A modification of the AIC is suggested by Hurvich and Tsai (1989) for situations where the sample size is small in relation to the number of fitted parameters. This modification, the corrected AIC (AIC_c), is calculated as follows:

$$AIC_c = -2 \log \left(\lambda \left(\hat{\theta} \mid y \right) \right) + 2K \left(\frac{n}{n-K-1} \right) \qquad (7.32)$$

where n is the sample size and all other terms are as in (7.31). In general, unless the sample size is large in relation to the number of estimated parameters, (7.32) is preferred over (7.31).

To illustrate, non-linear discriminant analysis was applied to the British cattle TB data. The dataset used included records of all TB outbreaks (i.e. 482, 0.01 degree resolution image pixels containing one or more TB outbreaks, representing disease presence) and a sample of 3,000 non-outbreak farms (representing disease absence). Environmental data were extracted for each presence or absence location, and the entire presence or absence data set was clustered using the k-means clustering algorithm of the SPSS statistical package (SPSS Inc. Chicago, Illinois) to produce five presence and five absence clusters. This entire dataset (presence and absence) was sampled randomly, with replacement, 100 times to generate sub-samples, each consisting of 300 records of presence and 300 records of absence. Each sub-sample was modelled using stepwise inclusion of variables from the environmental predictor database up to a maximum of 10 variables. The selection criterion was to maximize kappa or the AUC_c at each step. Once a set of predictor variables was chosen it was used with the input imagery to generate posterior probability predictions that each image pixel belonged to the presence group. The 100 images were then averaged to produce a single output image (Fig. 7.14). There was little difference between the predictions using the two different variable selection criteria, so only the AUC predictions are shown in Fig. 7.14.

The average value of the AUC for the 100 models averaged in Fig. 7.14 was 0.94 (SD 0.014). The top ten models in the series (sorted on AUC values) had an average AUC of 0.95 (SD 0.003) and the bottom ten an average of 0.92 (SD 0.006). For comparison, the three equivalent figures for the kappa statistic were 0.71 (SD 0.036), 0.76 (SD 0.016), and 0.66 (SD 0.024) respectively. The kappa values suggest that the models provided good to excellent fits to the data (Landis and Koch 1977).

The key environmental variables producing these fits are themselves quite variable. A commonly chosen variable is the tri-annual phase of air temperature (selected first in the 'best' model). Another is the bi-annual amplitude of the VPD (not selected at all in the best model, but frequently selected in the rest). In our experience these components of the higher Fourier harmonics generally operate to modulate the expression of the dominant annual cycle either by extending or curtailing the length of the season, or by changing the shape of the annual seasonal profile from pure sinusoidal to either flat-topped or more-peaked seasonality.

The analyses summarized in Fig. 7.14 take no account of the spatial arrangement of the infected farms. If there is a chance of contagion of one pixel from another, by virtue of its proximity rather than its environmental conditions, then further steps should be added to the analyses and model predictions. Generally a Gibbs sampler routine is applied but this slows down the modelling process considerably (each model is produced iteratively, for what is often a relatively modest increase in model accuracy (Rogers 2006)).

7.8 Conclusions

In this chapter an overview of the techniques that may be used to quantify the effect that explanatory variables have on the spatial distribution of an outcome of interest is provided. It was shown how accounting for spatial dependence provides at least two useful benefits in terms of enhancing understanding of the factors associated with the distribution of disease. Firstly, the regression coefficients from models that account for spatial dependence are less precise (compared with those that ignore it) meaning that the null hypothesis is less likely to be rejected when it is true (a Type I error). Secondly, mapping the structured heterogeneity terms from models that account for spatial dependence provides an indication of where disease risk is unaccounted for by the parameterized fixed effects, which can indicate where to look for previously unrecognized factors influencing the occurrence of disease.

The subject of spatial statistics is rapidly evolving with considerable progress made in recent years in the development of methodologies related to disease mapping and ecological analyses, particularly in the fields of multilevel modelling and Bayesian statistics. With the increasing availability of data (particularly that which has been remotely sensed), analytical techniques, high speed computers, and user-friendly software it is likely that researchers will seek to develop increasingly sophisticated models in an effort to refine their understanding of the behaviour of diseases in human and animal populations. While this is tangible evidence of progress, the enthusiasm with which these techniques are applied needs to be

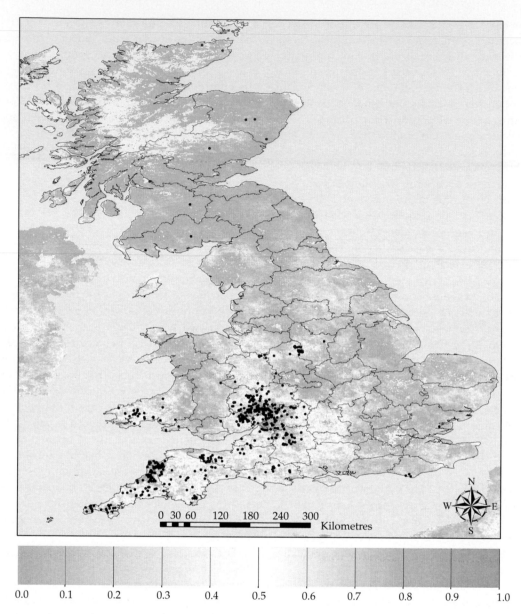

Figure 7.14 Mean (of 100) posterior probability risk map of bovine tuberculosis (TB) cases in Great Britain predicted by discriminant analytical models using step-wise inclusion of 10 variables to maximize the area under the curve (AUC) at each step. Five presence and five absence clusters were used for each bootstrap sample of 300 presence and 300 absence points sampled at random, with replacements, from a population of 482 presence and 3000 absence pixels (a presence pixel is a 0.01 degree pixel with at least one TB-positive farm in 1997; an absence pixel has farms, but no TB-positive ones in the same period). Posterior probability is on the green to red colour scale shown in the legend beneath the figure. The positive pixels are indicated by the black dots. See plate 10.

balanced with due consideration to factors such as data quality, the robustness of the chosen methods to misspecification, and the need for model validation. In this respect, spatial modelling is best conducted as an iterative process in which a research question is posed, data collected, a model developed, and uncertainty quantified, which should in turn guide further (focused) collection of data and model refinement. Other (no less important) issues are related to study design in situations where data are to be collected prospectively, rather than opportunistically, and choice of analytical techniques appropriate for the resolution, nature, and quality of the data at hand.

CHAPTER 8

Spatial risk assessment and management of disease

8.1 Introduction

The effective detection and control of diseases in humans and animals by health authorities needs to take into account spatial patterns of the disease's occurrence and any associated risk factors. This includes efficient data collection, management, and analysis. The integration of GIS functionality into most modern disease information systems reflects recognition of the importance of the spatial dimension of disease control. The analytical functionality of such systems is typically restricted to producing descriptive maps, often based on aggregations of data at the level of some administrative area, such as district or province. As a result of recent disease emergencies such as severe acute respiratory syndrome (SARS), FMD, and avian influenza, decision makers are now looking for tools that make more effective use of the wide range of available data sources, including analytical and modelling methods (Carpenter and Ward 2003; Lawson and Kleinman 2005b) in an attempt to increase our ability to detect unusual occurrences of disease and to allow for targeted surveillance and control efforts that account explicitly for spatial variation in risk.

When applying spatial analysis methods as part of disease management rather than as a research tool, the outputs need to be interpreted with some caution, particularly due to potential errors and biases (Neutra 1999; Elliott and Wakefield 2000; Jacquez 2004). For example, cluster detection methods may have a significant chance of turning up false positive results as well as having limited statistical power (Wakefield et al. 2000). In a research context, the users of such results are duly cautious,

but in an operational, planning context users may be less aware of, and less competent at evaluating, such potential pit-falls

The information that decision makers expect to obtain from risk assessments includes the level of disease risk and information on important risk factors, particularly if these can be influenced as part of risk mitigation. To prevent misinterpretation, the estimates of risk should always be accompanied by explicit statements about their uncertainty, and the potential influence of biases. It is important to recognize that the resulting risk management procedures are also influenced by other considerations such as political factors and societal values.

8.2 Spatial data in disease risk assessment

Spatial methods can be used to assess risks within the context of disease risk analysis, and thus help decision makers to develop risk management strategies. Disease risk assessments require some level of understanding of the underlying causal processes, as well as access to a range of data sources. The most basic data needed would be georeferenced, quantitative information about disease occurrence and the population at risk. These data can often be complemented by various types of risk factor data such as attributes of potentially at-risk individuals or groups, their contact networks, or environmental information (Boscoe et al. 2004).

Disease status information can be collected using targeted or scanning surveillance. The former is aimed at defining levels of, or absence of disease in specific populations, and the latter at maintaining a continuous watch for the occurrence of known and unknown diseases. Targeted surveillance is based on structured, cross-sectional, or longitudinal data collection approaches and may involve assessment of all, or a sample of, the individuals or groups potentially at risk. It typically includes the collection of denominator data as well as disease data. In contrast, scanning surveillance uses disease reporting information collected by health professionals as part of their routine job, or by farmers and other members of the public when they identify such diseases, or indicators thereof, such as dead birds (West Nile virus) or dead badgers (bovine TB). This means that the data are subject to varying degrees, of reporting bias and do not include denominator information. Both surveillance methods have been a standard component of disease management for a long time, but have tended to be inadequately georeferenced for the purpose of advanced spatial analysis. This has changed as a result of, for example, the availability of digital address databases and GPS.

The main focus of disease surveillance data is usually to record disease status information which, if combined with population at risk data, allows visualization of the spatial pattern of disease risk. The higher the spatial resolution of the data for a given area, the higher the statistical power for detecting events that occur in small regions (Lawson and Kleinman 2005b). More complex analyses aimed at explaining the variation in risk require access to risk factor information, which may be collected as part of targeted surveillance activities or may be accessed by linking surveillance data to census information or other risk factors such as environmental information. Depending on the type of link, this requires either database queries in database management software or spatial overlay operations in a GIS.

A fairly recent development has been the collation of network data in many European countries, in particular those that record the movements of individual animals among farms, livestock markets, and slaughterhouses (Klovdahl 2005; Webb 2005). A new development in landscape ecology has been the quantification of landscape structure (Gustafson 1998; McGarigal 2002). The resulting metrics can then be used as attribute information for risk assessments. They are particularly useful if wildlife densities are an important risk factor. For example, the density of some wild animal species may be higher in a landscape containing a large number of relatively small patches of forest, compared to one with a single contiguous forest patch of the same total area. This difference between habitats can be expressed as average patch size for each landscape. The public domain software Fragstats[44] allows the calculation of such metrics (McGarigal and Marks 1995).

All the data sources mentioned above are affected by some degree of bias. This may affect attribute information such as disease diagnosis or risk factor data, or it can be bias associated with the spatial reference. The choice of the sample selection method and the spatial resolution at which the data are collected will both result in sampling error in the attribute data

Syndromic surveillance is a new methodology that has been developed in response to a perceived need for early warning of bioterrorism attacks (Lawson and Kleinman 2005b). It does not monitor specific disease outcomes, but rather events that are indicative of the occurrence of diseases such as emergency room complaints, ambulance dispatch data, clinical diagnosis data, private over-the-counter and prescription medication sales, nurse help-line telephone logs, and absenteeism in schools (Miller et al. 2004b). It can also use spatial information as demonstrated by Heffernan et al. (2004) and Kulldorff et al. (2005). One of the problems with syndromic surveillance is the high risk of false positive alarms and the resulting cost of follow-up investigations (Fienberg and Shmueli 2005). For example, based on a pre-test probability of 0.0014 for anthrax and a very high assumed detection sensitivity/specificity of the surveillance system of 99%, Bravata et al. (2004) estimate that only 12% of the positive system responses would be true anthrax cases.

8.3 Spatial analysis in disease risk assessment

The spatial analysis tools suitable for risk assessment include the whole range of methods from

---

[44] http://www.umass.edu/landeco/research/fragstats/fragstats.html

visualization through to modelling techniques. The modelling techniques can be categorized into data-driven and knowledge-driven methods. The former is characterized by the use of statistical methods for defining relationships between risk factors and disease risk as the outcome variable, while knowledge-driven modelling approaches are based on existing knowledge about the causal relationships associated with the disease risk of interest.

8.4 Data-driven models of disease risk

As described above, statistical analysis is used to generate data-driven models from information collected through surveillance and other means. Spatial dependence can be accommodated using the methods described in Chapter 7. Such models generate quantitative estimates of risk and the relative weights of risk factors. There is a perception that these models are more valid than knowledge-based ones due to the apparently more objective method of defining the relationships. However, it needs to be emphasized that they are strongly dependent on the quality of the data and the validity of the model in the context of a particular decision problem. It is to be noted that Bayesian modelling approaches introduce prior knowledge to a data-driven approach, in that informative priors can be used for which the distributional characteristics are usually defined based on existing knowledge.

While the extent of bias associated with model predictions needs to be presented in a qualitative commentary, the statistical uncertainty associated with the outputs from such models should be presented together with the predicted risk estimates. For example, this can be done by presenting maps of the risk estimates together with maps of some specified upper and lower confidence limits.

In addition, decision makers need to be given aids that allow predictions to be transferred into their particular decision context. Often this means deciding on an appropriate course of action, such as whether or not to vaccinate in selected geographical areas. This decision should be based on localized risk estimates and their uncertainty, and then on the risk threshold above which populations in the respective areas should be vaccinated.

The choice of such thresholds should be associated with a risk of misclassifying the area based on the model prediction, which is influenced by the model validity. The statistical aspects of this relationship (not the bias) can be expressed as the model prediction's sensitivity and specificity for any given threshold, which can be presented very effectively using a ROC curve (Pfeiffer 2004).

Fig. 8.1 presents an example of this approach (Pfeiffer et al. 1997) in which a mixed effects logistic regression analysis was conducted to produce a map predicting the risk of East Coast fever outbreaks (caused by the protozoal haemoparasite *Theileria parva*), in cattle in Zimbabwe (Fig. 8.1a). The parasite occurs in East Africa, and as it includes the brown ear tick, *Rhipicephalus appendiculatus*, in

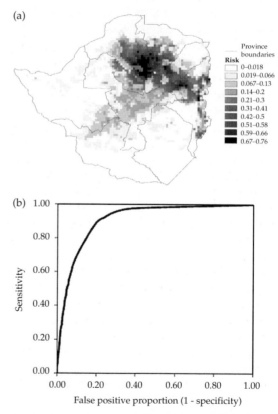

Figure 8.1 Risk map for theileriosis occurrence risk in Zimbabwe (Pfeiffer et al. 1997). a) Map showing probability of occurrence of outbreaks due to infection with *Theileria parva* and b) the ROC curve for the logistic regression model used to produce the risk map. Reproduced from Pfeiffer et al. (1997).

Table 8.1 Probability cut-off values associated with the ROC curve presented in Figure 8.1. Reproduced from Pfeiffer et al. (1997)

Cut-off	Sensitivity	Specificity	False positive proportion
0	1.00	0.00	1.00
0.02	0.98	0.62	0.38
0.06	0.93	0.76	0.24
0.1	0.85	0.83	0.17
0.16	0.69	0.90	0.10
0.22	0.61	0.93	0.07
0.32	0.50	0.95	0.05
0.42	0.40	0.96	0.04
0.46	0.35	0.97	0.03
0.54	0.25	0.98	0.02
0.64	0.12	0.99	0.01
0.74	0.01	1.00	0.00

its life cycle, environmental factors can be used to predict the spatial pattern of disease occurrence. The resulting risk map can, for example, be used to identify potential areas for vaccination by selecting a cut-off for outbreak risk, and vaccinating in all areas above that value. The ROC curve presented in Fig. 8.1b summarizes the fit of the model, but can also be used to identify an appropriate cut-off value. One of the criteria for this decision could be the likelihood of vaccinating in an area that is likely to be a false positive (x-axis in Fig. 8.1b) weighed against the likelihood of not vaccinating in an area where outbreaks may occur (y-axis in Fig. 8.1b). The shape of the ROC curve suggests that if resources are scarce, and therefore vaccinating false positives should be avoided, choosing a cut-off greater than or equal to 0.32 will result in 50% of those areas at risk of outbreaks being vaccinated and thereby being protected. On the other hand, 5% of those areas that are not at risk of outbreaks will also be vaccinated, resulting in wasted resources. Table 8.1 shows the probability cut-off values associated with the ROC curve presented in Fig. 8.1b.

8.5 Knowledge-driven models of disease risk

As an alternative to data-driven models, qualitative or quantitative risk estimates can be produced based on existing or hypothesized understanding of the causal relationships leading to disease occurrence. This type of model is not useful for identifying risk factors, as *a priori* knowledge about these and their interrelationships are used to define the model. Data-driven models are usually based on statistical regression models that include proxy risk factor variables associated with unobserved disease transmission processes. A strength of the knowledge-driven approach is that transmission dynamics can be modelled directly in that the changes in infection status of herds or individuals are represented. Disadvantages can be that the models become rather theoretical, have a strong subjective element, and are only loosely connected to real data. Models generated using this approach may be static or dynamic. Static models are defined as sets of linked rules of attribute information combined to produce risk estimates. Dynamic models reproduce patterns of change in time and space with respect to disease status in a population as a result of specified spatial and attribute factors.

8.5.1 Static knowledge-driven models

The basic principle of static knowledge-driven models is to define a set of weighted rules based on existing published and/or expert knowledge (Bonham-Carter 1994; Chrisman 2003). The simplest approach combines Boolean geographical overlays that reflect defined threshold values for decision criteria using Boolean logic with conjunctive (AND) or disjunctive (OR) operators. However, whether or not a given alternative satisfies a specific criterion may not be clearly defined. A number of methods have been developed to deal with this kind of uncertainty, such as Bayesian inference, fuzzy logic, and Dempster-Shafer theory (DST), all of which have been applied in a general decision-making context as well as in spatial decision-making.

Fuzzy logic can be used to model uncertainty where the possibility of a criterion being satisfied is defined on a continuous scale by a 'membership function' which can be rectilinear, sigmoidal, exponential, or any other shape. If there are multiple criteria for determining suitability, a method needs to be adopted to combine the criteria. One such method is weighted linear combination (WLC) in which criteria are standardized for comparison on a common scale and then weights applied to each criterion so that more important criteria exert a greater influence on the outcome. Finally, a weighted average across criteria is calculated for each alternative (or spatial unit), giving the final suitability estimate. This methodology can be implemented through multicriteria decision analysis (MCDA). Although fuzzy logic, implemented within a WLC framework, has been applied to assist MCDA in a wide range of spatial settings, animal health applications have rarely been reported. Examples include prioritizing areas for insect vector control (Robinson et al. 2002) and spatial modelling of tick vectors (Estrada-Peña 1997). Fuzzy logic models have also been used to determine the suitability of regions in Africa for malaria (Snow et al. 1998; 1999) and Rift Valley fever (Clements et al. 2006c).

DST (Dempster 1966; 1967) is a generalization of Bayes theory that is thought more accurately to represent uncertainty in near-ignorance situations (Luo and Caselton 1997). Uncertainty can be any known or unknown error, ambiguity or variation in a decision process, or can refer to the data on which the decision process is based (Eastman 2001). Uncertainty in geographical data may lead to erroneous decisions and subsequent adverse consequences. Eastman (2001) states that,

> 'although considerable attention has been paid to the issue of uncertainty, the manner in which uncertainties combine to affect the decision process and decision risk has received less interest.'

In the DST framework, probabilities may be assigned in the form of basic probability assignments (BPA) to unions of intervals or individual values in addition to the intervals/values themselves, and this allows for a much more flexible approach to uncertainty representation. The *belief* (the lower bound of probability) that the true value lies within a certain interval (or has a certain value), is calculated as the sum of the probability values assigned to that interval (or value) and to subsets of that interval. The *plausibility* (the upper bound of probability) that the true value lies within a given interval (or equals a given value) is calculated as the complement of the sum of probability values for intervals that exclude that interval or value. The difference

between plausibility and belief (termed the 'belief interval' by Eastman (2001)) represents the level of uncertainty surrounding true probability.

There is an increasing number of reports of DST applications. Examples include Sadiq and Rodriguez (2005), who use DST to examine water quality data and Luo and Caselton (1997) who apply DST to an analysis of climate change uncertainties. Clements et al. (2006c) use DST to identify areas in Senegal suitable for Rift Valley fever infection. However, there is a dearth of applications in epidemiological or health-related settings, particularly in a spatial context. Currently, approximations of belief functions, analogous to empirical Bayes estimation, are used in DST applications although computational advances may lead to full implementation of DST in the future (Haenni and Lehmann 2003).

MCDA, also known as multicriteria decision-making (MCDM), involves a sequence of analytical steps: (1) defining the objective(s); (2) defining the factors (continuous) and constraints (Boolean); (3) defining the relationship between each factor and suitability; (4) standardizing the factors so that they can be compared; (5) defining the relative importance of each factor in relation to the objective; (6) combining all factors and constraints to produce a final weighted estimate of suitability for each location in the study area; (7) sensitivity analysis; and (8) map validation.

A commonly-used method for integrating factors and constraints is WLC. There are a number of sources of information that may be utilized to determine the weights for WLC and the BPA in DST, such as statistical data, published literature, or expert opinion (Robinson et al. 2002; Osei-Bryson 2003). It may be necessary to take account of non-compensation among the factors, for instance, if a high score for one factor should not be offset by a low score for another factor due to some biological, or other, reason. This can be done using ordered weighted averaging (OWA) rather than WLC, where the factors are weighted for a given pixel according to the rank of their suitability scores within that pixel (Jiang and Eastman 2000). For a less compensatory model, lower ranked factors are given a higher relative weight. Uncertainty in the decision process arises from a number of sources including measurement error, inherent variability, conceptual ambiguity, or ignorance of model parameters.

A number of common pitfalls in the application of WLC are discussed by Malczewski (2000), who states that the attributes (i.e. factors and constraints) should be measurable and complete (i.e. cover all relevant aspects of the decision problem). Factor selection based on data availability is criticized. However, comprehensive data on a number of important disease factors are not always available and it often remains necessary to select attributes from limited available data resources. Correlation among attributes is also highlighted as an important issue by Malczewski (2000) who refers to this as a redundancy problem that gives rise to double-counting. The issue of spatial scale and levels of aggregation (MAUP) are also highlighted by Malczewski (2000). Other issues raised by the same author are attribute linearity, where transformation of the attribute for subsequent comparison does not take into account possible non linear associations with suitability, and incorrect weighting as a result of failing to consider the unit of measurement and range of the attribute.

The following example uses the British cattle TB data to illustrate how MCDA might be used in an epidemiological setting. It is assumed that wildlife reservoirs, particularly badgers, are partly responsible for the high prevalence of TB in certain parts of England and Wales. As badgers are known to have very specific requirements when choosing a site for their sett, the hypothesis for this example was that areas with a high prevalence of TB corresponded to areas most suitable for the construction of badger setts. The GIS software IDRISI was used to implement the model as it has a decision-support module for performing MCDA.

Following the hypothesis stated above, the objective of this MCDA model was to identify areas in England and Wales suitable for the construction of badger setts. A review of the relevant literature identified the criteria that influence where badgers build their setts (and therefore the criteria that needed to be included in the model) as being soil-type, landcover, and proximity to a food source. The literature revealed that setts are generally located in woodland, with broadleaf being greatly preferred to coniferous woodland, on well-drained soils and close to pastures (in which earthworms, the badger's staple diet, abound). As setts are only located on well-drained soils this criterion was included in the model as a constraint (Boolean) and the three landcover criteria (broadleaf woodland, coniferous woodland, and pasture) were included as factors (continuous). Each criterion was represented as a raster map layer (Fig. 8.2).

Factors were weighted using the pairwise comparison method (Saaty 1980), in which each factor is rated according to its relationship with each of the others, and weights were calculated for each factor based on this pairwise rating (Table 8.2). As the units and scales of the factor maps varied, the maps were standardized by converting each scale to a 0–255 byte binary scale, and then combined using WLC, resulting in a map in which each pixel (representing 1 km^2) was classified as either low, medium, or high, according to its degree of suitability for sett construction (Fig. 8.3a). The model identified, among other areas, the south and south-west of England and most of Wales to be moderately to highly suitable for badger sett construction, as well as the parts of East Anglia and Cumbria. Sensitivity analysis, which involves varying the weights of the factors and measuring the average change in the suitability scores at 10,000 randomly selected locations on the map, revealed little change in the suitability estimates.

In an epidemiological situation, validation of the resulting maps is not always possible due to lack of data, and is frequently limited to visual comparisons with existing data sources (Craig et al. 1999; Clements et al. 2006c). The most appropriate way to validate the map in Fig. 8.3a would be to overlay the actual locations of badger setts in order to determine whether high numbers of setts occur in those areas identified by the model as being most suitable for sett construction and *vice versa*. However, in the absence of data on sett locations, and given the hypothesis, an overlay of the 1996 TB high risk areas in England and Wales was used to indirectly validate the suitability map (Fig. 8.3b). The overlay was created from Fig. 6.2c (by drawing around those areas on the map with a high TB risk). This overlay showed a reasonable match with areas considered to be suitable for badger setts (south and south-west of England, parts of Wales, and Cumbria), but some pockets of high TB risk occur in areas that are apparently unsuitable for sett construction,

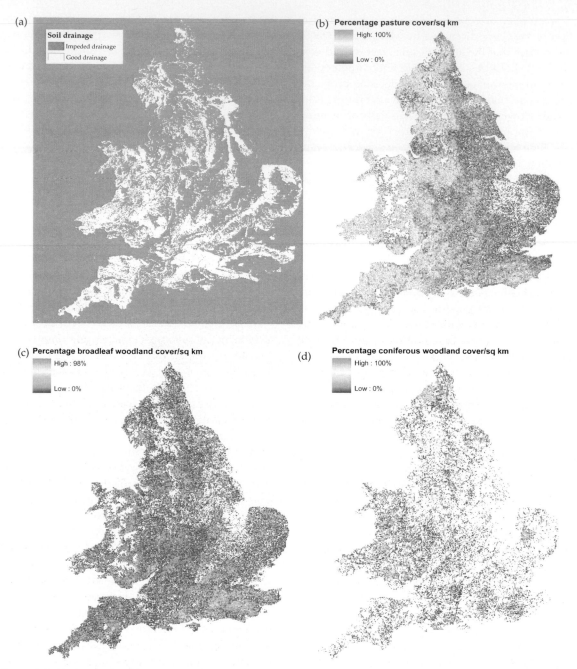

Figure 8.2 Criterion maps used in the MCDA model. (a) Boolean map showing soils with good or impeded drainage, (b) a continuous scale map of pasture in England and Wales (percentage cover/km²), (c) a continuous scale map of broadleaf woodland in England and Wales (percentage cover/km²), and (d) a continuous scale map of coniferous woodland in England and Wales (percentage cover/km²). See plate 11.

Table 8.2 Pairwise comparison matrix and calculated weights of factors for the location of badger setts

	Broadleaf	Coniferous	Pasture	Weight
Broadleaf	**1**	5	1	0.4806
Coniferous	1/5	**1**	1/3	0.1140
Pasture	1	3	**1**	0.4054

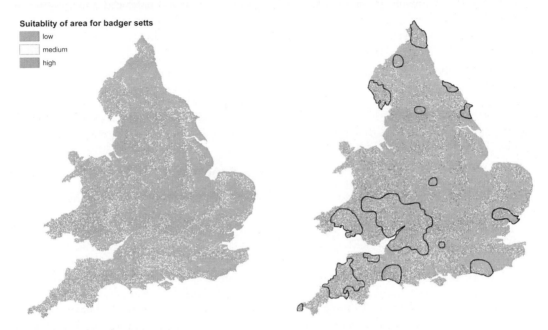

Suitablity of area for badger setts
- low
- medium
- high

Figure 8.3 (a) Map identifying areas in England and Wales of low, medium, and high suitabililty for the construction of badger setts, and (b) the suitability map with an overlay of the 1996 TB high-risk areas in England and Wales. See plate 12.

suggesting that factors other than badgers, such as cattle movement, may contribute to the high risk of TB in areas modelled as being unsuitable for sett construction.

8.5.2 Dynamic knowledge-driven models

Examination of the possible behaviour of infectious diseases, either in relation to the implementation of different disease control interventions or following their hypothetical introduction into populations, requires models that can represent the dynamics of the disease, often primarily in time, but which can also include a spatial dimension. The modelling approaches range from highly aggregated

models, such as susceptible-infected-recovered (SIR) type mathematical models, to very detailed simulations explicitly representing events affecting individual farms, households, or persons.

To keep the models as simple as possible, the majority still focus mainly on the temporal dimension of population and infection dynamics, thereby minimizing both the computing resources needed and the necessary level of detailed understanding of the epidemiological mechanisms involved. However, a trend has recently developed for models to be more complex and also spatially explicit. This allows transmission mechanisms associated with geographical proximity and environmental factors to be represented, but also makes significant demands with respect to the quantitative knowledge about the epidemiology of an infection.

Modelling methodologies have become more advanced during the last 10 years, facilitated by the availability of more powerful computers, and supported by an increased demand from risk managers for predictive information on the progression of a disease and the impact of potential control methods. Unfortunately, for many diseases the necessary data concerning the epidemiological relationships underlying the relevant infection's temporal and spatial dynamics are still inadequate. It is therefore of paramount importance that these dynamic knowledge-driven models are validated and peer-reviewed before they are used to inform decision making.

An epidemiological example of dynamic knowledge-driven modelling is presented in Savill et al. (2006). When developing a mathematical model of the spread of FMD in Great Britain in 2001 they incorporate distance between farms, and between farms and roads. They suggest that this relatively simple spatial representation allows effective aggregated representation of several transmission mechanisms. Morris et al. (2001) simulate the impact of different control strategies during the same outbreak of FMD using a Monte Carlo approach where the geographical location of farms and livestock markets, and the resulting interactions relevant to virus spread, are explicitly incorporated in the model structure. This allows for the separate representation of four different transmission mechanisms namely, movement of animals for trade purposes, local spread to nearby farms, long-distance windborne spread, and spread through dairy tanker movements.

A recent development is the inclusion of the contact structure of populations at risk (Keeling and Eames 2005; Kao et al. 2006). While this is not necessarily a spatial representation, it focuses on direct contact as a possible transmission mechanism, which is itself partly influenced by geographical proximity. Eubank et al. (2004) developed a simulation model of a smallpox outbreak for an urban population of 1.5 million people, in which the daily activities resulting in the opportunity for transmission of the disease are represented using a social network structure. Gilbert et al. (2005) show that

inclusion of data on animal movements from the United Kingdom's cattle tracking database greatly increases the power of a model to predict TB breakdowns, over environmental factors alone.

The outputs from dynamic spatial models can be effectively communicated using maps, as shown by Ferguson et al. (2006) who present avian influenza risk amongst humans in Great Britain and the USA. Keeling et al. (2001) produced a map movie depicting the simulated temporal and spatial spread of FMD during the UK 2001 epidemic, which can be downloaded via the journal's website[45]. It needs to be emphasized that such maps should be accompanied by appropriate commentary that explains the assumptions behind the models, and therefore allows consideration of the potential biases and uncertainties reflected in the map.

8.6 Conclusion

The inclusion of spatial models in the process of risk assessment and management has become increasingly common over the last 10 years. This has been made possible through advances in computer hardware and software, the development of appropriate analytical algorithms, and the availability of a multitude of databases, many of which are georeferenced. In addition, there has been an increasing demand for evidence-based decision making which includes the need to produce spatially explicit inferences. Models have much potential to assist in decision making but are also associated with many risks and, due to the often complex calculations involved, outputs are often viewed with some scepticism by decision makers. The increasing use of knowledge- as well as data-driven approaches opens up many opportunities, not only for research but also for policy development. It has to be noted that although the tools may have advanced in sophistication and the data quantity increased exponentially, data quality has not improved at the same rate, and when developing knowledge-driven models it usually becomes apparent that our knowledge of basic biological mechanisms remains deficient. So while models, including those that are spatially explicit, allow gaps in the existing knowledge to

---

[45] http://www.sciencemag.org

be identified, they also provide significant opportunities for enhancing our understanding of the underlying epidemiological processes, as well as allowing the key pieces of information that should become the focus of research to be defined. A particular strength of the spatial dimension is that spatial model outputs can be visualized through maps, greatly facilitating effective communication. However, an implicit danger is that while risk managers are often impressed by the visualizations, they may in fact underestimate the influence of biases and uncertainty in relation to the data and epidemiological mechanisms. Additional emphasis therefore needs to be placed on recognizing and communicating bias and uncertainty, and in this context in particular, static knowledge-driven modelling approaches provide a set of effective, yet underutilized, tools.

References

Aamodt, G., Samuelsen, S.O., Skrondal, A., 2006. A simulation study of three methods for detecting disease clusters. *International Journal of Health Geographics* **5**, 15.

Abernethy, D.A., Pfeiffer, D.U., Denny, G.O.O., Torrens, T.D., McCullough, S.J., Graham, D.A., 2000. Evaluating airborne spread in a Newcastle disease epidemic in Northern Ireland. In: Salman, M., Morley, P., and Ruch-Gallie, R. (Eds.), *Proceedings of the 9th Symposium of the International Society for Veterinary Epidemiology and Economics*. Breckenridge, Colorado, USA, August 7–11.

Abrial, D., Calavas, D., Lauvergne, N., Morignat, E., Ducrot, C., 2003. Descriptive spatial analysis of BSE in western France. *Veterinary Research* **34**, 749–760.

Abrial, D., Calavas, D., Jarrige, N., Ducrot, C., 2005. Spatial heterogeneity of the risk of BSE in France following the ban of meat and bone meal in cattle feed. *Preventive Veterinary Medicine* **67**, 69–82.

Akaike, H., 1973. Information theory as an extension of the maximum likelihood principle. In: Petrov, B.N. and Csaki, F. (Eds.), *Second International Symposium on Information Theory*, pp. 267–281. Akademiai Kiado, Budapest.

Alexander, F.E., Boyle, P., 2000. Do cancers cluster?, In: Elliott, P., Wakefield, J.C., Best, N.G., Brigs, D.J. (Eds.), *Spatial Epidemiology*, pp. 302–316. Oxford University Press, Oxford.

Alexander, F.E., Cuzick, J., 1992. Methods for the assessment of disease clusters. In: Elliott, P., Cuzick, J., English, D., Stern, R. (Eds.), *Geographical and Environmental Epidemiology: Methods for Small-Area Studies*, pp. 238–250. Oxford University Press, Oxford.

Alexander, F.E., Williams, J., McKinney, P.A., Ricketts, T.J., Cartwright, R.A., 1989. A specialist leukaemia/lymphoma registry in the UK. Part 2: Clustering of Hodgkin's disease. *British Journal of Cancer* **60**, 948–952.

Alexander, F.E., Ricketts, T.J., Williams, J., Cartwright, R.A., 1991. Methods of mapping and identifying small clusters of rare diseases with applications in geographical epidemiology. *Geographical Analysis* **23**, 158–173.

Ali, M., Goovaerts, P., Nazia, N., Haq, M.Z., Yunus, M., Emch, M., 2006. Application of Poisson kriging to the mapping of cholera and dysentery incidence in an endemic area of Bangladesh. *International Journal of Health Geographics* **5**, 45.

Anselin, L., 1995. Local indicators of spatial association – LISA. *Geographical Analysis* **27**, 93–115.

Anselin, L., 1996. The Moran scatterplot as an ESDA tool to assess local instability in spatial association., In: Fischer, M., Scholten, H., Unwin, D. (Eds.), *Spatial Analytical Perspectives on GIS*, pp. 111–125. Taylor and Francis, London.

Anselin, L., Syabri, I., Kho, Y., 2006. GeoDa: An introduction to spatial data analysis. *Geographical Analysis* **38**, 5–22.

Antunes, J., Waldman, E., 2002. Trends and spatial distribution of deaths of children aged 12–60 months in Sao Paulo, Brazil, 1980–98. *Bulletin of the World Health Organization* **80**, 391–398.

Arlinghaus, S., 1995. *Practical Handbook of Spatial Statistics*. CRC Press, New York.

Armitage, P., Berry, G., Mathews, J., 2002. *Statistical Methods in Medical Research*. Blackwell Publications, London.

Baddeley, A., Turner, R., 2000. Practical maximum pseudolikelihood for spatial point patterns (with discussion). *Australian and New Zealand Journal of Statistics* **43**, 283–322.

Baddeley, A., Turner, R., 2002. Spatstat – Analysis for spatial point patterns. http://www.spatstat.org.

Bailey, T.C., Gatrell, A.C., 1995. *Interactive Spatial Data Analysis*. Longman Group, Harlow.

Baker, R.D., 1996. Testing for space-time clusters of unknown size. *Journal of Applied Statistics* **23**, 543–554.

Banerjee, S., Carlin, B.P., Gelfand, A.E., 2004. *Hierarchical Modelling and Analysis of Spatial Data*. Chapman & Hall/CRC Press, USA.

Bartlett, M.S., 1947. Multivariate analysis. *Journal of the Royal Statistical Society, Series B* **9**, 176–197.

Barton, D.E., David, F.N., Merrington, M., 1965. A criterion for testing contagion in time and space. *Annals of Human Genetics* **29**, 97–103.

Bell, B.S., Hoskins, R., Pickle, L., Wartenberg, D., 2006. Current practices in spatial analysis of cancer data: mapping health statistics to inform policymakers and the public. *International Journal of Health Geographics* **5**, 49.

Bellec, S., Hemon, D., Rudant, J., Goubin, A., Clavel, J., 2006. Spatial and space-time clustering of childhood acute leukaemia in France from 1990 to 2000: a nationwide study. *British Journal of Cancer* **94**, 763–770.

Bellido, J., Pierce, G., Wang, J., 2001. Modelling intra-annual variation in abundance of squid *Loligo forbesi* in Scottish waters using generalised additive models. *Fisheries Research* **52**, 23–39.

Benardinelli, L., Clayton, D., Montomoli, C., 1995. Bayesian estimates of disease maps: How important are priors? *Statistics in Medicine* **14**, 2411–2431.

Berke, O., 2004. Exploratory disease mapping: kriging the spatial risk function from regional count data. *International Journal of Health Geographics* **3**, 18.

Berman, M., Turner, T., 1992. Approximating point process likelihoods with GLM. *Applied Statistics* **41**, 31–38.

Besag, J., 1989. Towards Bayesian image analysis. *Journal of Applied Statistics* **16**, 395–407.

Besag, J., Mollié, A., 1989. Bayesian mapping of mortality rates. *Bulletin of the International Statistical Institute* **53**, 127–128.

Besag, J., Newell, J., 1991. The detection of clusters in rare diseases. *Journal of the Royal Statistical Society, Series A* **154**, 143–155.

Besag, J., York, J., Mollié, A., 1991. Bayesian image restoration with two applications in spatial statistics. *Annals of the Institute of Statistics and Mathematics* **43**, 1–59.

Best, N., Waller, L., Thomas, A., Conlon, E., Arnold, R., 1999. Bayesian models for spatially correlated disease and exposure data. In: Bernardo, J., Berger, J., Dawid, A., Smith, A. (Eds.), *Bayesian Statistics 6: Proceedings of the Sixth Valencia Meeting on Bayesian Statistics.* pp. 131– 156, Oxford University Press, Oxford.

Best, N., Ickstadt, K., Wolpert, R., 2000. Spatial Poisson regression for health and exposure data measured at disparate resolutions. *Journal of the American Statistical Association* **95**, 1076–1088.

Best, N., Richardson, S., Thomson, A., 2005. A comparison of Bayesian spatial models for disease mapping. *Statistical Methods in Medical Research* **14**, 35–59.

Bithell, J.F., 1990. An application of density estimation to geographical epidemiology. *Statistics in Medicine* **9**, 691–701.

Bithell, J.F., 1995. The choice of test for detecting a raised disease risk near a point source. *Statistics in Medicine* **14**, 2309–2322.

Bithell, J.F., Stone, R.A., 1989. On statistical methods for analysing the geographical distribution of cancer cases near nuclear installations. *Journal of Epidemiology and Community Health* **43**, 79–85.

Bithell, J.F., Dutton, S.J., Draper, G.J., Neary, N.M., 1994. Distribution of childhood leukaemias and non-Hodgkin's lymphomas near nuclear installations in England and Wales. *British Medical Journal* **309**, 501–505.

Black, D. 1984. *Investigation of the Possible Increased Incidence of Cancer in West Cumbria.* Her Majesty's Stationary Office, London.

Böhning, D., Schlattmann, P., 1992. Computer-assisted analysis of mixtures (CAMAN): Statistical algorithms. *Biometrics* **48**, 283–303.

Bonetti, M., Pagano, M., 2004. The interpoint distance distribution as a descriptor of point patterns with an application to spatial disease clustering. *Statistics in Medicine* **24**, 753–773.

Bonham-Carter, G.F., 1994. *Geographic Information Systems for Geoscientists: Modelling with GIS.* Elsevier Science, Oxford.

Borchers, D., Buckland, S., Priede, I., Ahmadi, S., 1997. Improving the precision of the daily egg production method using generalised additive models. *Canadian Journal of Fish and Aquatic Sciences* **54**, 2727–2742.

Boscoe, F.P., McLaughlin, C., Schymura, M.J., Kielb, C.L., 2003. Visualization of the spatial scan statistic using nested circles. *Health and Place* **9**, 273–277.

Boscoe, F., Ward, M., Reynolds, P., 2004. Current practices in spatial analysis of cancer data: data characteristics and data sources for geographic studies of cancer. *International Journal of Health Geographics* **3**, 28.

Bowman, A.W., Azzalini, A., 1997. *Applied Smoothing Techniques for Data Analysis: The Kernel Approach with S-Plus Illustrations.* Oxford University Press, Oxford.

Bravata, D.M., Sundaram, V., McDonald, K.M., Smith, W.M., Szeto, H., Schleinitz, M.D., Owens, D.K., 2004. Evaluating detection and diagnostic decision support systems for bioterrorism response. *Emerging Infectious Diseases* **10**, 100–108.

Breslow, N., Clayton, D., 1993. Approximate inference in generalised linear mixed models. *Journal of the American Statistical Association* **88**, 9–25.

Breslow, N., Day, N., 1987. The *Design and Analysis of Cohort Studies Volume 2,* IARC Scientific Publication No. 82. International Agency for Research on Cancer, Lyon.

Breusch, T., Pagan, A., 1979. A simple test for heteroscedasticity and random coefficient variation. *Econometrica* **47**, 1287–1294.

Broman, A.T., Shun, K., Munoz, B., Duncan, D.D., West, S.K., 2006. Spatial clustering of ocular chlamydial infection over time following treatment, among households in a village in Tanzania. *Investigative Ophthalmology and Visual Science* **47**, 99–104.

Brooker, S., Clarke, S., Njagi, J.K., Polack, S., Mugo, B., Estambale, B., Muchiri, E., Magnussen, P., Cox, J., 2004. Spatial clustering of malaria and associated risk factors during an epidemic in a highland area of western Kenya. *Tropical Medicine and International Health 9*, 757–766.

Browne, W., 2005. *MCMC Estimation in MLwiN Version 2.0*. Centre for Multilevel Modelling, University of Bristol, Bristol.

Buntinx, F., Geys, H., Lousbergh, D., Broeders, G., Cloes, E., Dhollander, D., Op De Beeck, L., Vanden Brande, J., Van Waes, A., Molenberghs, G., 2003. Geographical differences in cancer incidence in the Belgian province of Limburg. *European Journal of Cancer* **39**, 2058–2072.

Burra, T., Jerrett, M., Burnett, R.T., Anderson, M., 2002. Conceptual and practical issues in the detection of local disease clusters: A study of mortality in Hamilton, Ontario. *The Canadian Geographer 46*, 160–171.

Burrough, P.A., McDonnell, R.A., 1998. *Principles of Geographical Information Systems*. Oxford University Press, Oxford.

Caldwell, G.G., 1990. Twenty-two years of cancer cluster investigations at the centers for disease control. *American Journal of Epidemiology 132*, S43–S47.

Canters, F., DeClair, H., 1989. *The World in Perspective: A Directory of World Map Projections*. John Wiley & Sons, Chichester.

Carpenter, T.E., Ward, M.P., 2003. Methods for determining spatial clusters in surveillance and survey programs. In: Salman, M.D. (Ed.), *Animal Disease Surveillance and Survey Systems*, pp. 101–117, Iowa State University Press, Iowa.

Carpenter, T.E., Chriel, M., Andersen, M.M., Wulfson, L., Jensen, A.M., Houe, H., Greiner, M., 2006. An epidemiologic study of late-term abortions in dairy cattle in Denmark, July 2000-August 2003. *Preventive Veterinary Medicine 77*, 215–229.

Carr, D., Wallin, J., Carr, D., 2000. Two new templates for epidemiology applications: Linked micromap plots and conditioned choropleth maps. *Statistics in Medicine* **19**, 2521–2538.

Carrat, F., Valleron, A.-J., 1992. Epidemiologic mapping using the "Kriging" method: application to an influenza-like illness epidemic in France. *American Journal of Epidemiology* **135**, 1293–1300.

CDC, 1990. Guidelines for investigating clusters of health events. *MMWR* **39** (RR-11), 1–16.

Chalmers, A.F., 1999. *What Is This Thing Called Science?* Open University Press, Buckingham.

Chaput, E.K., Meek, J.I., Heimer, R., 2002. Spatial analysis of human granulocytic ehrlichiosis near Lyme, Connecticut. *Emerging Infectious Diseases 8*, 943–948.

Chetwynd, A.G., Diggle, P.J., 1998. On estimating the reduced second moment measure of a stationary spatial point process. *Australian and New Zealand Journal of Statistics* **40**, 11–15.

Chrisman, N., 2003. *Exploring Geographic Information Systems*. John Wiley & Sons, New York.

Christensen, O., Ribeiro Jr, P., Diggle, P., 2002. geoRglm. *R News* **2**, 26–28.

Clayton, D., Bernardinelli, L., 1992. Bayesian methods for mapping disease risk. In: Elliott, P., Cuzick, J., English, D., Stern, R. (Eds), *Geographical and Environmental Epidemiology: Methods for Small-Area Studies*, pp. 205–220. Oxford University Press, Oxford.

Clayton, D., Kaldor, J., 1987. Empirical Bayes estimates of age-standardized relative risks for use in disease mapping. *Biometrics 43*, 671–681.

Clements, A.C., Pfeiffer, D.U., Otte, M.J., Morteo, K., Chen, L., 2002. A global livestock production and health atlas (GLiPHA) for interactive presentation, integration and analysis of livestock data. *Preventive Veterinary Medicine* **56**, 19–32.

Clements, A., Lwambo, N., Blair, L., Nyandindi, U., Kaatano, G., Kinung'hi, S., Webster, J., Fenwick, A., Brooke, S., 2006a. Bayesian spatial analysis and disease mapping: tools to enhance planning and implementation of a schistosomiasis control programme in Tanzania. *Tropical Medicine and International Health* **11**, 490–503.

Clements, A., Moyeed, R., Brooker, S., 2006b. Bayesian geostatistical prediction of the intensity of infection with *Schistosoma mansoni* in East Africa. *Parasitology*, **133**, 711–719.

Clements, A.C.A., Pfeiffer, D.U., Martin, V., 2006c. Application of knowledge-driven spatial modelling approaches and uncertainty management to a study of Rift Valley fever in Africa. *International Journal of Health Geographics* **5**, 57.

Cliff, A., 1995a. Analysing geographically related disease data. *Statistical Methods in Medical Research* **4**, 93–101.

Cliff, A.D. (Ed.), 1995b. Special Issue: Analysing geographically-related disease data. *Statistical Methods in Medical Research* 4, 93–184.

Cliff, A.D., Ord, J.K., 1973. *Spatial Autocorrelation*. Pion Limited, London.

Cliff, A.D., Ord, J.K., 1981. *Spatial Processes: Models and Applications*. Pion Limited, London.

Congdon, P., 2003. *Applied Bayesian Modelling*. John Wiley & Sons, Chichester.

Conlon, E., Louis, T., 1999. Addressing multiple goals in evaluating region specific risk using Bayesian methods. In: Lawson, A., Biggeri, A., Böhning, D., Lesaffre, E., Viel, J.-F., Bertollini, R. (Eds.), *Disease Mapping and Risk Assessment for Public Health*, pp. 31–47. John Wiley, London.

Cousens, S., Smith, P.G., Ward, H., Everington, D., Knight, R.S.G., Zeidler, M., Stewart, G., Smith-Bathgate, E.A.B., Macleod, M.-A., Mackenzie, J., Will, R.G., 2001. Geographical distribution of variant Creutzfeldt-Jakob disease in Great Britain, 1994-2000. *Lancet* **357**, 1002–1007.

Craig, M.H., Snow, R.W., Le Sueur, D., 1999. A climate-based distribution model of malaria transmission in sub-Saharan Africa. *Parasitology Today* **15**, 105–111.

Cressie, N., 1992. Smoothing regional maps using empirical Bayes predictors. *Geographical Analysis* **24**, 75–95.

Cressie, N.A.C., 1993. *Statistics for Spatial Data*. John Wiley & Sons, New York.

Cromley, E., McLafferty, S., 2002. *GIS and Public Health*. The Guilford Press, New York.

Cuzick, J., Edwards, R., 1990. Spatial clustering for inhomogeneous populations (with discussion). *Journal of the Royal Statistical Society Series B* **52**, 73–104.

Dempster, A.P., 1966. New methods for reasoning towards posterior distributions based on sample data. *Annals of Mathematical Statistics* **37**, 355–374.

Dempster, A.P., 1967. Upper and lower probabilities induced by a multivalued mapping. *Annals of Mathematical Statistics* **38**, 325–339.

Devine, O., Louis, T., Halloran, M., 1994a. Empirical Bayes estimators for spatially correlated incidence rates. *Environmetrics* **5**, 381–398.

Devine, O., Louis, T., Halloran, M., 1994b. Empirical Bayes methods for stabilising incidence rates before mapping. *Epidemiology* **5**, 622–630.

Diggle, P., 1990. A point process modelling approach to raised incidence of a rare phenomenon in the vicinity of a prespecified point. *Journal of the Royal Statistical Society Series A* **153**, 349–362.

Diggle, P.J., 2000. Overview of statistical methods for disease mapping and its relationship to cluster detection. In: Elliott, P., Wakefield, J.C., Best, N.G., Briggs, D.J. (Eds.), *Spatial Epidemiology – Methods and Applications*, pp. 87–103. Oxford University Press, Oxford.

Diggle, P.J., 2003. *Statistical Analysis of Spatial Point Patterns*. Arnold Publishers, London.

Diggle, P., Chetwynd, A., 1991. Second order analysis of spatial clustering for inhomogeneous populations. *Biometrics* **47**, 1155–1163.

Diggle, P., Elliott, P., 1995. Disease risk near point sources: Statistical issues in the analysis of disease risk near point sources using individually or spatially aggregated data. *Journal of Epidemiology and Community Health* **49**, S20 –S27.

Diggle, P., Ribeiro Jr, P., 2007. *Model-based Geostatistics*. Springer Science, New York.

Diggle, P., Rowlingson, B., 1994. A conditional approach to point process modelling of elevated risk. *Journal of the Royal Statistical Society Series A (Statistics in Society)* **157**, 433–440.

Diggle, P.J., Tawn, J.A., 1998. Model-based geostatistics. *Applied Statistics* **47**, 299–350.

Diggle, P.J., Chetwynd, A.G., Häggkvist, R., Morris, S.E., 1995. Second-order analysis of space-time clustering. *Statistical Methods in Medical Research* **4**, 124–136.

Diggle, P., Morris, S., Morton-Jones, T., 1999. Case-control isotonic regression for investigation of elevation in risk around a point source. *Statistics in Medicine* **18**, 1605–1613.

Diggle, P., Moyeed, R., Rowlingson, B., Thomson, M., 2002. Childhood malaria in the Gambia: A case study in model-based geostatistics. *Journal of the Royal Statistical Society Series C (Applied Statistics)* **51**, 493–506.

Ding, Y., Fotheringham, A.S., 1992. The integration of spatial analysis and GIS. *Computers in Environmental and Urban Systems* **16**, 3–19.

Doherr, M.G., Zurbriggen, A., Hett, A.R., Rufenacht, J., Heim, D., 2002. Geographical clustering of cases of bovine spongiform encephalopathy (BSE) born in Switzerland after the feed ban. *The Veterinary Record* **151**, 467–472.

Dolk, H., Elliott, P., Shaddick, G., Walls, P., Thakrar, B., 1997a. Cancer incidence near radio and television transmitters in Great Britain. II: All high power transmitters. *American Journal of Epidemiology* **145**, 10–17.

Dolk, H., Shaddick, G., Walls, P., Grundy, C., Thakrar, B., Kleinschmidt, I., Elliott, P., 1997b. Cancer incidence near radio and television transmitters in Great Britain. I: Sutton Coldfield transmitter. *American Journal of Epidemiology* **145**, 1–9.

Doll, S.R., 1989. The epidemiology of childhood leukaemia. *Journal of the Royal Statistical Society Series A* **152**, 341–351.

Dorling, D., 1995. The visualization of local urban change across Britain. *Environment and Planning B: Planning and Design* **22**, 269–290.

Drijver, M., Melse, J.M., 1992. Disease clusters and environmental contamination. I: a guide for public health services. *T Soc Gezondheidsz* **70**, 565–570.

Duczmal, L., Assunção, R., 2004. A simulated annealing strategy for the detection of arbitrarily shaped spatial clusters. *Computational Statistics and Data Analysis* **45**, 269–286.

Duczmal, L., Kulldorff, M., Huang, L., 2006. Evaluation of spatial scan statistics for irregularly shaped disease clusters. *Journal of Computational and Graphical Statistics.* **15**, 428–442.

Durr, P.A., Froggatt, A.E., 2002. How best to geo-reference farms? A case study from Cornwall, England. *Preventive Veterinary Medicine* **56**, 51–62.

Durr, P., Gatrell, A., 2004. *GIS and Spatial Analysis in Veterinary Science.* CABI Publishing, Wallingford.

Dwass, M., 1957. Modified randomization tests for non-parametric hypotheses. *The Annals of Mathematical Statistics* **28**, 181–187.

Eastman, J.R., 2001. *Guide to GIS and Image Processing.* Clark Labs, Clark University, Worcester, MA.

Ederer, F., Myers, M.H., Mantel, N., 1964. A statistical problem in space and time: Do leukaemia cases come in clusters? *Biometrics* **20**, 626–638.

Ekstrand, C., Carpenter, T.E., 1998. Spatial aspects of foot-pad dermatitis in Swedish broilers. *Acta Veterinaria Scandinavica* **38**, 278–280.

Elliott, P., Wakefield, J.C., 2000. Bias and confounding in spatial epidemiology. In: Elliott, P., Wakefield, J.C., Best, N.G., Briggs, D.J. (Eds.), *Spatial Epidemiology – Methods and Applications,* pp. 68–84. Oxford University Press, Oxford.

Elliott, P., Wakefield, J., 2001. Disease clusters: Should they be investigated, and, if so, when and how? *Journal of the Royal Statistical Society: Series A* **164**, 3–12.

Elliott, P., Wartenberg, D., 2004. Spatial epidemiology: current approaches and future challenges. *Environmental Health Perspectives* **112**, 998–1006.

Elliott, P., Cuzick, J., English, D., Stern, R., 1992a. *Geographical & Environmental Epidemiology – Methods for Small-Area Studies.* Oxford University Press, Oxford.

Elliott, P., Hills, M., Beresford, J., Kleinschmidt, I., Jolley, D., Pattenden, S., Rodrigues, L., Westlake, A., Rose, G., 1992b. Incidence of cancers of the larynx and lung near incinerators of waste solvents and oils in Great Britain. *The Lancet* **339**, 854–859.

Elliott, P., Martuzzi, M., Shaddick, G., 1995. Spatial statistical methods in environmental epidemiology: A critique. *Statistical Methods in Medical Research* **4**, 137–159.

Elliott, P., Shaddick, G., Kleinschmidt, I., Jolley, D., Walls, P., Beresford, J., Grundy, C., 1996. Cancer incidence near municipal solid waste incinerators in Great Britain. *British Journal of Cancer* **73**, 702–710.

Elliott, P., Wakefield, J.C., Best, N.G., Briggs, D.J., 2000. *Spatial Epidemiology – Methods and Applications.* Oxford University Press, Oxford.

Estrada-Peña, A., 1997. Epidemiological surveillance of tick populations: a model to predict the colonization success of *Ixodes ricinus* (Acari: Ixodidae). *European Journal of Epidemiology* **13**, 573–580.

Eubank, S., Guclu, H., Kumar, V.S., Marathe, M.V., Srinivasan, A., Toroczkai, Z., Wang, N., 2004. Modelling disease outbreaks in realistic urban social networks. *Nature* **429**, 180–184.

Falconi, F., Ochs, H., Deplazes, P., 2002. Serological cross-sectional survey of psoroptic sheep scab in Switzerland. *Veterinary Parasitology* **109**, 119–127.

Fang, Z., Kulldorff, M., Gregorio, D.I., 2004. Brain cancer mortality in the United States, 1986 to 1995: a geographic analysis. *Neuro-Oncology* **6**, 179–187.

Ferguson, N.M., Cummings, D.A.T., Fraser, C., Cajka, J.C., Cooley, P.C., Burke, D.S., 2006. Strategies for mitigating an influenza pandemic. *Nature* **443**, 448–452.

Fevre, E.M., Coleman, P.G., Odiit, M., Magona, J.W., Welburn, S.C., Woolhouse, M.E.J., 2001. The origins of a new *Trypanosoma brucei rhodesiense* sleeping sickness outbreak in eastern Uganda. *The Lancet* **358**, 625–628.

Fienberg, S.E., Shmueli, G., 2005. Statistical issues and challenges associated with rapid detection of bioterrorist attacks. *Statistics in Medicine* **24**, 513–529.

Fischer, G., van Velthuizen, H., Shah, M., Nachtergaele, F., 2002. *Global Agro-Ecological Assessment for Agriculture in the 21st Century: Methodology and Results.* Research Report RR-02-02. Laxenburg: International Institute for Applied Systems Analysis and Food and Agriculture Organisation of the United Nations.

Forand, S.P., Talbot, T.O., Druschel, C., Cross, P.K., 2002. Data quality and the spatial analysis of disease rates: Congenital malformations in New York State. *Health and Place* **8**, 191–199.

Fortin, M.-J., Jacquez, G.M., 2000. Randomization tests and spatially autocorrelated data. *Bulletin of the Ecological Society of America* **81**, 201–205.

Fosgate, G.T., Carpenter, T.E., Chomel, B.B., Case, J.T., DeBoss, E.E., Reilly, K.F., 2002. Time-space clustering of human brucellosis, California, 1973-1991. *Emerging Infectious Diseases* **8**, 672–678.

Fotheringham, A.S., Zhan, F.B., 1996. A comparison of three exploratory methods for cluster detection in spatial point patterns. *Geographical Analysis* **28**, 200–218.

French, N.P., Berriatua, E., Wall, R., Smith, K.L., Morgan, K.L., 1999. Sheep scab outbreaks in Great Britain between 1973 and 1992: Spatial and temporal patterns. *Veterinary Parasitology* **83**, 187–200.

French, N.P., McCarthy, H.E., Diggle, P.J., Proudman, C.J., 2005. Clustering of equine grass sickness cases in the United Kingdom: A study considering the effect of position-dependent reporting on the space-time K-function. *Epidemiology and Infection* **133**, 343–348.

Gardner, M.J., 1989. Review of reported increases of childhood cancer rates in the vicinity of nuclear installations in the UK. *Journal of the Royal Statistical Society Series A* **152**, 307–325.

Gardner, M.J., 1992. Childhood leukaemia around the Sellafield nuclear plant. In: Elliott, P., Cuzick, J., English, D., Stern, R. (Eds.), *Geographical and Environmental Epidemiology: Methods for Small-Area Studies*, pp. 209–309. Oxford University Press, Oxford.

Gatrell, A., Bailey, T., 1996. Interactive spatial data analysis in medical geography. *Social Science and Medicine* **42**, 843–855.

Gatrell, A.C., Löytönen, M., 1998. *GIS and Health*. Taylor & Francis, London.

Gay, E., Senoussi, R., Barnouin, J., 2007. A spatial hazard model for cluster detection on continuous indicators of disease: Application to somatic cell score. *Veterinary Research* **38**, 585–596.

Geary, R., 1954. The contiguity ratio and statistical mapping. *The Incorporated Statistician* 5, 115–145.

Gelman, A.B., Carlin, J.S., Stern, H.S., Rubin, D.B. 1995. *Bayesian Data Analysis*, p. 526. Chapman & Hall/CRC, Boca Raton, Florida.

George, M., Wiklund, L., Aastrup, M., Pousette, J., Thunholm, B., Saldeen, T., Wernroth, L., Zarén, B., Holmberg, L., 2001. Incidence and geographical distribution of sudden infant death syndrome in relation to content of nitrate in drinking water and ground water levels. *European Journal of Clinical Investigation* **31**, 1083–1094.

Getis, A., Ord, J.K., 1992. The analysis of spatial association by use of distance statistics. *Geographical Analysis* **24**, 189–206.

Getis, A., Ord, J.K., 1996. Local spatial statistics: An overview. In: Longley, P., Batty, M. (Eds.), *Spatial Analysis: Modelling in a GIS Environment*, pp. 261-277. Geoinformation International, Cambridge,

Getis, A., Ord, J.K., 1998. The use of a local statistic to study the diffusion of AIDS from San Francisco. In: Griffith, D.A., Amrhein, C.G., Huriót, J.-M. (Eds.), *Econometric Advances in Spatial Modelling and Methodology: Essays in Honour of Jean Paelinck*, pp. 143–158. Kluwer, Dordrecht.

Ghosh, M., Natarajan, K., Stroud, T., Carlin, B., 1998. Generalized linear models for small-area estimation. *Journal of the American Statistical Association* **93**, 273–282.

Gilbert, E.W., 1958. Pioneer maps of health and disease in England. *Geographical Journal* **124**, 172–183.

Gilbert, M., Mitchell, A., Bourn, D., Mawdsley, J., Clifton-Hadley, R., Wint, W., 2005. Cattle movements and bovine tuberculosis in Great Britain. *Nature* **435**, 491–496.

Goetz, S.J., Prince, S.D., Small, J., 2000. Advances in satellite remote sensing of environmental variables for epidemiological applications. *Advances in Parasitology* **47**, 289–307.

Goldstein, H., 1995. *Multilevel Statistical Models*. Edward Arnold, London.

Goovaerts, P., 2006. Geostatistical analysis of disease data: accounting for spatial support and population density in the isopleth mapping of cancer mortality risk using area-to-point Poisson kriging. *International Journal of Health Geographics* **5**, 52.

Gotway, C., 2004. *Statistical Methods for Spatial Data Analysis*. Chapman & Hall/CRC Press, New York, USA.

Gotway, C.A., Wolfinger, R.D., 2003. Spatial prediction of counts and rates. *Statistics in Medicine* **22**, 1415–1432.

Graham, S.L., Barling, K.S., Waghela, S., Scott, H.M., Thompson, J.A., 2005. Spatial distribution of antibodies to *Salmonella enterica* serovar Typhimurium O antigens in bulk milk from Texas dairy herds. *Preventive Veterinary Medicine* **69**, 53–61.

Green, P.E., 1978. *Analyzing Multivariate Data*. The Dryden Press, Illinois..

Green, R.M., Hay, S.I., 2002. The potential of Pathfinder AVHRR data for providing surrogates of climatic variables across Africa and Europe for epidemiological applications. *Remote Sensing of Environment* **79**, 165–175.

Green, C., Hoppa, R.D., Young, T.K., Blanchard, J.F., 2003. Geographic analysis of diabetes prevalence in an urban area. *Social Science and Medicine* **57**, 551–560.

Gregorio, D.I., Samociuk, H., 2003. Breast cancer surveillance using gridded population units, Connecticut, 1992 to 1995. *Annals of Epidemiology* **13**, 42–49.

Grimson, R., Wang, K., Johnson, P., 1981. Searching for hierarchical clusters of disease: Spatial patterns of sudden infant death syndrome. *Society for Science in Medicine* **15D**, 287–293.

Gustafson, E.J., 1998. Quantifying landscape spatial pattern: what is the state of the art? *Ecosystems* **1**, 143–156.

Haenni, R., Lehmann, N., 2003. Implementing belief function computations. *International Journal of Intelligent Systems* **18**, 31–49.

Haining, R., 2003. *Spatial Data Analysis – Theory and Practice*. Cambridge University Press, Cambridge, UK.

Haining, R., Wise, S., Ma, J., 1998. Exploratory spatial data analysis in a geographic information systems environment. *The Statistician* **47**, 457–469.

Hammond, R., McGrath, G., Martin, S., 2001. Irish soil and land-use classifications as predictors of numbers of badgers and badger setts. *Preventive Veterinary Medicine* **51**, 137–148.

Hanchette, C., Schwartz, G., 1992. Geographic patterns of prostate-cancer mortality. Evidence for a protective effect of ultraviolet-radiation. *Cancer* **70**, 2861–2869.

Hanson, C.E., Wieczorek, W.F., 2002. Alcohol mortality: a comparison of spatial clustering methods. *Social Science and Medicine* **55**, 791–802.

Haslett, J., Bradley, R., Craig, P., Unwin, A., Wills, G., 1991. Dynamic graphics for exploring spatial data with application to locating global and local anomalies. *The American Statistician* **45**, 234–242.

Hastie, T., Tibshirani, R., 1990. *Generalised Additive Models.* Chapman and Hall, London.

Hay, S.I., 2000. An overview of remote sensing and geodesy for epidemiology and public health application. *Advances in Parasitology* **47**, 1–35.

Hay, S.I., Lennon, J.J., 1999. Deriving meteorological variables across Africa for the study and control of vector-borne disease: a comparison of remote sensing and spatial interpolation of climate. *Tropical Medicine and International Health* **4**, 58–71.

Hay, S.I., Graham, A., Rogers, D.J., 2006. *Global Mapping of Infectious Diseases: Methods, Examples and Emerging Applications.* Academic Press, Amsterdam.

Haybittle, J., Yuen, P., Machin, D., 1995. Multiple comparisons in disease mapping. *Statistics in Medicine* **14**, 2503–2505.

Heffernan, R., Mostashari, F., Das, D., Karpati, A., Kulldorff, M., Weiss, D., 2004. Syndromic surveillance in public health practice, New York City. *Emerging Infectious Diseases* **10**, 858–864.

Henderson, T.W., 1990. Toxic tort litigation: Medical and scientific principles in causation. *American Journal of Epidemiology* **132**, S69–S78.

Hills, M., Alexander, F., 1989. Statistical methods used in assessing the risk of disease near a source of possible environmental pollution: A review. *Journal of the Royal Statistical Society Series A* **152**, 353–363.

Hjalmars, U., Kulldorff, M., Gustafsson, G., Nagarawalla, N., 1996. Childhood leukaemia in Sweden: Using GIS and a spatial scan statistic for cluster detection. *Statistics in Medicine* **15**, 707–715.

Hjalmars, U., Kulldorff, M., Wahlqvist, Y., Lannering, B., 1999. Increased incidence rates but no space-time clustering of childhood astrocytoma in Sweden, 1973-1992. *Cancer* **85**, 2077–2090.

Hoar, B.R., Chomel, B.B., Rolfe, D.L., Chang, C.C., Fritz, C.L., Sacks, B.N., Carpenter, T.E., 2003. Spatial analysis of *Yersinia pestis* and *Bartonella vinsonii* subsp *berkhoffii* seroprevalence in California coyotes (*Canis latrans*). *Preventive Veterinary Medicine* **56**, 299–311.

Huillard d'Aignaux, J., Cousens, S.N., Delasnerie-Lauprêtre, N., Brandel, J.-P., Salomon, D., Laplanche, J.-L., Hauw, J.-J., Alpérovitch, A., 2002. Analysis of the geographical distribution of sporadic Creutzfeldt-Jakob disease in France between 1992 and 1998. *International Journal of Epidemiology* **31**, 490–495.

Hurvich, C.M., Tsai, C.L., 1989. Regression and time series model selection in small samples. *Biometrika* **76**, 297–307.

Jacquez, G., 1994. Disease cluster statistics for imprecise space-time locations. *Statistics in Medicine* **15**, 873–885.

Jacquez, G., 1996. A *k* nearest neighbour test for space-time interaction. *Statistics in Medicine* **15**, 1935–1949.

Jacquez, G. 1998. GIS as an enabling technology. In: Gatrell, A., Löytönen, M. (Eds.), *GIS and Health,* pp. 17–28. Taylor & Francis, London.

Jacquez, G., 2004. Current practices in the spatial analysis of cancer: flies in the ointment. *International Journal of Health Geographics* **3**, 22.

Jacquez, G.M., Greiling, D.A., 2003. Local clustering in breast, lung and colorectal cancer in Long Island, New York. *International Journal of Health Geographics* **2**, 3.

Jacquez, G.M., Jacquez, J.A., 1999. Disease clustering for uncertain locations. In: Lawson, A., Biggeri, A., Böhning, D., Lesaffre, E., Viel, J.F., Bertollini, R. (Eds.), *Disease Mapping and Risk Assessment in Public Health,* pp. 151-168. John Wiley & Sons, Chichester.

Jacquez, G., Grimson, R., Kheifets, L., Waller, L., Wartenberg, D. (Eds.), 1992. Port Jefferson conference: Statistics and computing in disease clustering. *Statistics in Medicine* **12**, 1751–1968.

Jacquez, G., Grimson, R., Kheifets, L., Waller, L., Wartenberg, D., 1996. University of British Columbia conference: Statistics and computing in disease clustering. *Statistics in Medicine* **15**, 681–952.

Jarup, L., Best, N., Toledano, M., Wakefield, J., Elliott, P., 2002. Geographical epidemiology of prostate cancer in Great Britain. *International Journal of Cancer* **97**, 695–699.

Jemal, A., Kulldorff, M., Devesa, S.S., Hayes, R.B., Fraumeni Jr., J.F., 2002. A geographic analysis of prostate cancer mortality in the United States, 1970-89. *International Journal of Cancer* **101**, 168–174.

Jennings, J.M., Curriero, F.C., Celentano, D., Ellen, J.M., 2005. Geographic identification of high gonorrhea transmission areas in Baltimore, Maryland. *American Journal of Epidemiology* **161**, 73–80.

Jerrett, M., Burnett, R., Kanaroglou, P., Eyles, J., Finkelstein, N.G.C., Brook, J., 2001. A GIS-environmental justice analysis of particulate air pollution in Hamilton, Canada. *Environment and Planning A* **33**, 955–973.

Jiang, H., Eastman, J.R., 2000. Application of fuzzy measures in multi-criteria evaluation in GIS. *International Journal of Geographical Information Science* **14**, 173–184.

Neill, D.B., Moore, A.W., Cooper, G.F., 2006. A Bayesian scan statistic for spatial cluster detection. *Advances in Disease Surveillance* **1**, 55.

Neutra, R.R., 1999. Computer geographic analysis: A commentary of its use and misuse in public health. In: Lawson, A., Biggeri, A., Böhning, D., Lesaffre, E., Viel, J.F., Bertollini, R. (Eds.), *Disease Mapping and Risk Assessment for Public Health*, pp. 311–319. John Wiley & Sons, Chichester.

Nødtvedt, A., Guitian, J., Egenvall, A., Emanuelson, U., Pfeiffer, D.U., 2007. The spatial distribution of atopic dermatitis cases in a population of insured Swedish dogs. *Preventive Veterinary Medicine* **78**, 210–222.

Norström, M., Pfeiffer, D.U., Jarp, J., 2000. A space-time cluster investigation of an outbreak of acute respiratory disease in Norwegian cattle herds. *Preventive Veterinary Medicine* **47**, 107–119.

O'Brien, D.J., Kaneene, J.B., Getis, A., Lloyd, J.W., Swanson, G.M., Leader, R.W., 2000. Spatial and temporal comparison of selected cancers in dogs and humans, Michigan, USA, 1964-1994 *Preventive Veterinary Medicine* **47**, 187-204.

Oakes, M., 1986. *Statistical Inference*. John Wiley and Sons, Chichester.

Oden, N., 1995. Adjusting Moran's *I* for population density. *Statistics in Medicine* **14**, 17–26.

Olea-Popelka, F.J., Griffin, J.M., Collins, J.D., McGrath, G., Martin, S.W., 2003. Bovine tuberculosis in badgers in four areas in Ireland: Does tuberculosis cluster? *Preventive Veterinary Medicine* **59**, 103–111.

Olea-Popelka, F.J., Flynn, O., Costello, E., McGrath, G., Collins, J.D., O'Keeffe, J., Kelton, D.F., Berke, O., Martin, S.W., 2005. Spatial relationship between *Mycobacterium bovis* strains in cattle and badgers in four areas in Ireland. *Preventive Veterinary Medicine* **71**, 57–70.

Oliver, M.N., Smith, E., Siadaty, M., Hauck, F.R., Pickle, L.W., 2006. Spatial analysis of prostate cancer incidence and race in Virginia, 1990-1999. *American Journal of Preventive Medicine* **30**, S67–76.

Openshaw, S., 1984. *The Modifiable Areal Unit Problem* (Concepts and Techniques in Modern Geography, No. 38). Geo Books, Norwich.

Openshaw, S., Charlton, M., Wymer, C., Craft, A., 1987. A mark I geographical analysis machine for the automated analysis of point data sets. *International Journal of Geographical Information Systems* **1**, 335–358.

Openshaw, S., Craft, A., Charlton, M., Birch, J.M., 1988. Investigation of leukemia clusters by use of a geographical analysis machine. *Lancet* **1**, 272–273.

Openshaw, S., Cross, A., Charlton, M., 1990. Building a prototype geographical correlates exploration machine. *International Journal of Geographical Information Systems* **4**, 297–312.

Ord, J.K., Getis, A., 1993. Distributional issues concerning distance statistics. Working paper presented at the Annual Meeting of the North American Regional Science Association International, Houston, Texas.

Osei-Bryson, K.-M., 2003. Supporting knowledge elicitation and consensus building for Dempster-Shafer decision models. *International Journal of Intelligent Systems* **18**, 129–148.

Ozdenerol, E., Williams, B.L., Kang, S.Y., Magsumbol, M.S., 2005. Comparison of spatial scan statistic and spatial filtering in estimating low birth weight clusters. *International Journal of Health Geographics* **4**, 19.

Patil, G.P., Taillie, C., 2004. Upper level set scan statistic for detecting arbitrarily shaped hotspots. *Environmental and Ecological Statistics* **11**, 183–197.

Perez, A.M., Ward, M.P., Torres, P., Ritacco, V., 2002. Use of spatial statistics and monitoring data to identify clustering of bovine tuberculosis in Argentina. *Preventive Veterinary Medicine* **56**, 63–74.

Perneger, T.V., 1998. What's wrong with Bonferroni adjustments. *British Medical Journal* **316**, 1236–1238.

Perry, B., Kruska, R., Lessard, P., Norval, R., Kundert, K., 1991. Estimating the distribution and abundance of *Rhipicephalus appendiculatus* in Africa. *Preventive Veterinary Medicine* **11**, 261–268.

Pfeiffer, D.U., 2000. Spatial analysis – a new challenge for veterinary epidemiologists. In: Thrusfield, M.V., Goodall, E.A. (Eds.), *Proceedings of the Annual Meeting of the Society for Veterinary Epidemiology and Preventive Medicine, Edinburgh 29–31 March 2000*, pp. 86–106. Society for Veterinary Epidemiology and Preventive Medicine, Edinburgh.

Pfeiffer, D.U., 2004. Geographical information science and spatial analysis in animal health. In: Durr, P., Gatrell, A. (Eds.), *GIS and Spatial Analysis in Veterinary Science*, pp. 119–144. CABI Publishing, Wallingford.

Pfeiffer, D.U., Hugh-Jones, M., 2002. Geographical information systems as a tool in epidemiological assessment and wildlife disease management. *Revue Scientifique et Technique de l'Office International des Epizooties* **21**, 91–102.

Pfeiffer, D.U., Morris, R.S., 1994. Spatial analysis techniques in veterinary epidemiology. Rowlands, G.J., Kyule, M.N., and Perry, B.D. Special Issue: *Proceedings of the 7th International Symposium on Veterinary Epidemiology and Economics*, Nairobi, 15–19 August, 1994. *The Kenya Veterinarian* **18**, 483–485.

Pfeiffer, D.U., Duchateau, L., Kruska, R.L., Ushewokunze-Obatolu, U., Perry, B.D., 1997. A spatially predictive logistic regression model for occurrence of theileriosis outbreaks in Zimbabwe. *Epidemiologie et Santé Animale* **31–32**, 12.12.1–3.

Jones, R.C., Liberatore, M., Fernandez, J.R., Gerber, S.I., 2006. Use of a prospective space-time scan statistic to prioritize shigellosis case investigations in an urban jurisdiction. *Public Health Reports* **121**, 133–139.

Jung, I., Kulldorff, K., Klassen, A.C., 2006. A spatial scan statistic for ordinal data. *Statistics in Medicine* **26**, 1594–1607.

Kaluzny, S., Vega, S., Cardoso, T., Shelly, A., 1996. S+ SPATIALSTATS *User's Manual for Windows and Unix*. MathSoft, Inc Seattle, Washington.

Kao, R.R., Danon, L., Green, D.M., Kiss, I.Z., 2006. Demographic structure and pathogen dynamics on the network of livestock movements in Great Britain. *Proceedings of the Royal Society Series B* **273**, 1999–2007.

Keeling, M.J., Eames, K.T., 2005. Networks and epidemic models. *Journal of the Royal Society Interface* **2**, 295–307.

Keeling, M.J., Woolhouse, M.E.J., Shaw, D.J., Matthews, L., Chase-Topping, M., Haydon, D.T., Cornell, S.J., Kappey, J., Wilesmith, J., Grenfell, B.T., 2001. Dynamics of the 2001 UK foot and mouth epidemic: Stochastic dispersal in heterogeneous landscape. *Science* **294**, 813–817.

Kelsall, J.E., Diggle, P.J., 1995a. Kernel estimation of relative risk. *Bernoulli* **1**, 3–16.

Kelsall, J.E., Diggle, P.J., 1995b. Non-parametric estimation of spatial variation in relative risk. *Statistics in Medicine* **14**, 2335–2342.

Kelsall, J.E., Diggle, P.J., 1998. Spatial variation in risk: a nonparametric binary regression approach. *Applied Statistics* **47**, 559–573.

Kitron, U., Kazmierczak, J.J., 1997. Spatial analysis of the distribution of Lyme disease in Wisconsin. *American Journal of Epidemiology* **145**, 558–566.

Kitron, U., Michael, J., Swanson, J., Haramis, L., 1997. Spatial analysis of the distribution of Lacrosse Encephalitis in Illinois, using a geographic information system and local and global spatial statistics. *American Journal of Tropical Medicine and Hygiene* **57**, 469–475.

Klassen, A.C., Kulldorff, M., Curriero, F., 2005. Geographical clustering of prostate cancer grade and stage at diagnosis, before and after adjustment for risk factors. *International Journal of Health Geographics* **4**, 1.

Kleinman, K.P., Abrams, A.M., Kulldorff, M., Platt, R., 2005. A model-adjusted space-time scan statistic with an application to syndromic surveillance. *Epidemiology and Infection* **113**, 409–419.

Kleinschmidt, I., Sharp, B., Mueller, I., Vounatsou, P., 2002. Rise in malaria incidence rates in South Africa: A small-area spatial analysis of variation in time trends. *American Journal of Epidemiology* **155**, 257–264.

Klovdahl, A.S., 2005. Social network research and human subjects protection: Towards more effective infectious disease control. *Social Networks* **27**, 119–137.

Knox, E.G., 1989. Detection of clusters. In: Elliott, P. (Ed.) *Methodologies of Enquiry into Disease Clustering. Small Area*, Health Statistics Unit, pp. 17–22, London.

Knox, E.G., Bartlett, M.S., 1964. The detection of space-time interactions. *Applied Statistics* **13**, 25–30.

Knuesel, R., Segner, H., Wahli, T., 2003. A survey of viral diseases in farmed and feral salmonids in Switzerland. *Journal of Fish Diseases* **26**, 167–182.

Kreft, I., de Leeuw, J., 1998. *Introducing Multilevel Modelling*. Sage, London.

Krzanowski, W.J., Marriott, F.H.C., 1995. *Multivariate Analysis Part 2. Classification, Covariance Structures and Repeated Measurements*. Arnold, London.

Kulldorff, M., 1988. Statistical methods for spatial epidemiology: tests for randomness. In: Gatrell, A.C., Löytönen, M. (Eds.), *GIS and Health*, pp. 49–62. Taylor and Francis, London.

Kulldorff, M., 1997. A spatial scan statistic. *Communications in Statistics: Theory and Methods* **26**, 1481–1496.

Kulldorff, M., 1999. Statistical evaluation of disease cluster alarms. In: Lawson, A., Biggeri, A., Böhning, D., Lesaffre, E., Viel, J.F., Bertollini, R. (Eds.), *Disease Mapping and Risk Assessment in Public Health*, pp. 143–149. John Wiley & Sons, Chichester.

Kulldorff, M., 2001. Prospective time periodic geographical disease surveillance using a scan statistic. *Journal of the Royal Statistical Society Series A* **164**, 61–72.

Kulldorff, M. 2003. *SaTScan User Guide*. National Cancer Institute, Bethesda, MD.

Kulldorff, M., Hjalmars, U., 1999. The Knox method and other tests for space-time interaction. *Biometrics* **55**, 544–552.

Kulldorff, M., Nagarwalla, N., 1995. Spatial disease clusters: Detection and inference. *Statistics in Medicine* **14**, 799–819.

Kulldorff, M., Feuer, E.J., Miller, B.A., Freedman, L.S., 1997. Breast cancer clusters in the Northwest United States: A geographic analysis. *American Journal of Epidemiology* **146**, 161–170.

Kulldorff, M., Athas, W.F., Feuer, E.J., Miller, B.A., Key, C.R., 1998a. Evaluating cluster alarms: A space-time scan statistic and brain cancer in Los Alamos, New Mexico. *American Journal of Public Health* **88**, 1377–1380.

Kulldorff, M., Rand, K., Gherman, G., Williams, G., DeFrancesco, D. 1998b. *SaTScan: Software for the Spatial and Space-Time Scan Statistics*. National Cancer Institute, Bethesda, MD.

Kulldorff, M., Tango, T., Park, P.J., 2003. Power comparisons for disease clustering tests. *Computational Statistics and Data Analysis* **42**, 665–684.

Kulldorff, M., Heffernan, R., Hartman, J., Assuncao, R., Mostashari, F., 2005. A space-time permutation scan statistic for disease outbreak detection. *PLoS Medicine* **2**, e59.

Kulldorff, M., Song, C., Gregorio, D., Samociuk, H., DeChello, L., 2006a. Cancer map patterns: are they random or not? *American Journal of Preventive Medicine* **30**, S37–49.

Kulldorff, M., Huang, L., Pickle, L., Duczmal, L., 2006b. An elliptical spatial scan statistic. *Statistics in Medicine* **25**, 3929–3943.

Kyriakidis, P.C., 2004. A geostatistical framework for area-to-point spatial interpolation. *Geographical Analysis* **36**, 259–289.

Landis, J.R., Koch, G.C., 1977. The measurement of observer agreement for categorical data. *Biometrics* **33**, 159–174.

Lawson, A., 1989. Contribution to the `cancer near nuclear installations' meeting. *Journal of the Royal Statistical Society Series A* **152**, 374–375.

Lawson, A., 1992. GLIM and normalising constant models in spatial and directional data analysis. *Computational Statistics and Data Analysis* **13**, 331–348.

Lawson, A.B., 1993. On the analysis of mortality events associated with a prespecified fixed point. *Journal of the Royal Statistical Society Series A* **156**, 363–377.

Lawson, A., 1994. On using spatial Gaussian priors to model heterogeneity in environmental epidemiology. *Statistician* **43**, 69–76.

Lawson, A., 1995. MCMC methods for putative pollution source problems in environmental epidemiology. *Statistics in Medicine* **14**, 2473–2485.

Lawson, A.B., 2001a. *Statistical Methods in Spatial Epidemiology*. John Wiley & Sons, Chichester.

Lawson, A.B., 2001b. Disease map reconstruction. *Statistics in Medicine* **20**, 2183–2204.

Lawson, A.B., 2006a. *Statistical Methods in Spatial Epidemiology*, (2nd ed.). John Wiley & Sons, Chichester.

Lawson, A.B., 2006b. Disease cluster detection: A critique and a Bayesian proposal. *Statistics in Medicine* **25**, 897–916.

Lawson, A., Clark, A., 1999. Markov chain Monte Carlo methods for putative sources of hazard and general clustering. In: Lawson, A., Biggeri, A., Böhning, D., Lesaffre, E., Viel, J.-F., Bertollini, R. (Eds.), *Disease Mapping and Risk Assessment for Public Health*, pp. 119–142. John Wiley and Sons Ltd, London.

Lawson, A., Clark, A., 2002. Spatial mixture relative risk models applied to disease mapping. *Statistics in Medicine* **21**, 359–370.

Lawson, A.B., Denison, D.G.T., 2002. *Spatial Cluster Modelling*. Chapman & Hall/CRC Press, Boca Raton.

Lawson, A.B., Kleinman, K., 2005a. *Spatial and Syndromic Surveillance in Public Health*. John Wiley & Sons, Chichester.

Lawson, A.B., Kleinman, K., 2005b. Introduction: Spatial and syndromic surveillance for public health. In: Lawson, A.B., Kleinman, K. (Eds.), *Spatial and Syndromic Surveillance*, pp. 1–10. John Wiley & Sons, Chichester.

Lawson, A.B., Kulldorff, M., 1999. A review of cluster detection methods. In: Lawson, A., Biggeri, A., Böhning, D., Lesaffre, E., Viel, J.F., Bertollini, R. (Eds.), *Disease Mapping and Risk Assessment in Public Health*, pp. 143–149. John Wiley & Sons, Chichester.

Lawson, A.B., Williams, F.L.R., 1993. Applications of extraction mapping in environmental epidemiology. *Statistics in Medicine* **12**, 1249–1258.

Lawson, A., Williams, F., 1994. Armadale: A case study in environmental epidemiology. *Journal of the Royal Statistical Society Series A* **157**, 285–298.

Lawson, A.B., Williams, F.L.R., 2001. *An Introductory Guide to Disease Mapping*. John Wiley & Sons, Chichester.

Lawson, A.B., Waller, L.A., Biggeri, A., 1995. Special issue: Spatial disease patterns. *Statistics in Medicine* **14**, 2289–2508.

Lawson, A., Biggeri, A., Böhning, D., Lesaffre, E., Viel, J.F., Bertollini, R., 1999a. *Disease Mapping and Risk Assessment in Public Health*. John Wiley & Sons, Chichester.

Lawson, A.B., Biggeri, A., Dreassi, E., 1999b. Edge effects in disease mapping. In: Lawson, A., Biggeri, A., Böhning, D., Lesaffre, E., Viel, J.F., Bertollini, R. (Eds.), *Disease Mapping and Risk Assessment in Public Health*, pp. 83–96. John Wiley & Sons, Chichester.

Lawson, A.B., Browne, W.J., Vidal Rodeiro, C.L., 2003. *Disease Mapping with WinBUGS and MLwiN*. John Wiley & Sons, Ltd, Chichester

Le, N., Petkau, A., Rosychuk, R., 1996. Surveillance of clustering near point sources. *Statistics in Medicine* **15**, 727–740.

Legendre, P., Legendre, L., 1998. *Numerical Ecology*. Elsevier, Amsterdam.

Leiss, W., Powell, D., 2004. *Mad Cows and Mother's Milk*. McGill-Queen's University Press, Montreal & Kingston.

Leyland, A.H., Davies, C.A., 2005. Empirical Bayes methods for disease mapping. *Statistical Methods in Medical Research*. **14**, 17–34.

Leyland, A., Goldstein, H., 2001. *Multilevel Modelling of Health Statistics*. John Wiley & Sons, Ltd, Chichester.

Longley, P.A., Goodchild, M.F., Maguire, D.J., Rhind, D.W., 2001. *Geographic Information Systems and Science.*, Chichester.

Luo, W.B., Caselton, B., 1997. Using Dempster-Shafer theory to represent climate change uncertainties. *Journal of Environmental Management* **49**, 73–93.

Maheswaran, R., Strachan, D., Dodgeon, B., Best, N., 2002. A population-based case-control study for examining early life influences on geographical variation in adult mortality in England and Wales using stomach cancer and stroke as examples. *International Journal of Epidemiology* **31**, 375–382.

Malczewski, J., 2000. On the use of weighted linear combination method in GIS: common and best practice approaches. *Transactions in GIS* **4**, 5–22.

Mantel, N., 1967. The detection of disease clustering and a generalized regression approach. *Cancer Research* **27**, 209–220.

Manton, K., Woodbury, M., Stallard, E., 1981. A variance components approach to categorical data models with heterogenous mortality rates in North Carolina counties. *Biometrics* **37**, 259– 269.

Marcelo, C., Renato, A., 2005. A fair comparison between the spatial scan and Besag-Newell disease clustering tests. *Environmental and Ecological Statistics* **12**, 301–319.

Marshall, R.J., 1991a. A review of methods for the statistical analysis of spatial patterns of disease. *Journal of the Royal Statistical Society Series A* **154**, 421–441.

Marshall, R., 1991b. Mapping disease and mortality rates using empirical Bayes estimators. *Applied Statistics* **40**, 283–294.

McGarigal, K., 2002. Landscape pattern metrics. In: El-Shaarawi, A.H., Piegorsch, W.W. (Eds.), *Encyclopedia of Environmetrics Vol. 2*, pp. 1135–1142. John Wiley & Sons, Sussex.

McGarigal, K., Marks, B.J., 1995. *Fragstats: Spatial Pattern Analysis Program for Quantifying Landscape Structure*, p. 131. USDA Forest Service, Pacific Northwest Research Station, Portland.

McLeod, K.S., 2000. Our sense of Snow: the myth of John Snow in medical geography. *Social Science and Medicine* **50**, 923–935.

McPherson, J.M., Jetz, W., Rogers, D.J., 2004. The effects of species' range sizes on the accuracy of distribution models: ecological phenomenon or statistical artefact? *Journal of Applied Ecology* **41**, 811–823.

Meyers, R., Aramini, J., Lim, G., Stratton, J., Pollari, F., Sockett, P., Majowicz, S., 2002. Using Geographic Information Systems to identify the source of a waterborne gastrointestinal outbreak in Walkerton, Ontario, Canada, May–June, 2000. In: Rigby, J., Skelly, C., Wigham, P. (Eds.), *GeoHealth 2002 Proceedings of the Spatial Information Research Centre's 14th Colloquium* pp. 71–74. Victoria University, Wellington, New Zealand.

Michelozzi, P., Capon, A., Kirchmayer, U., Forastiere, F., Biggeri, A., Barca, A., Perlucci, C.A., 2002. Adult and childhood leukemia near a high-power radio station in Rome, Italy. *American Journal of Epidemiology* **155**, 1096–1103.

Miller, M.A., Gardner, I.A., Kreuder, C., Paradies, Worcester, K.R., Jessup, D.A., Dodd, E., Harris, Ames, J.A., Packham, A.E., Conrad, P.A., 2002. freshwater runoff is a risk factor for *Toxoplasm* infection of southern sea otters (*Enhydra lutri* *International Journal for Parasitology* **32**, 997–100

Miller, M.A., Grigg, M.E., Kreuder, C., Jam Melli, A.C., Crosbie, P.R., Jessup, D.A., Bo J.C., Brownstein, D., Conrad, P.A., 2004a. sual genotype of *Toxoplasma gondii* is cor California sea otters (*Enhydra lutris nereis*) cause of mortality. *International Journal for Pɪ* **34**, 275–284.

Miller, B., Kassenborg, H., Dunsmuir, W., (Hadidi, M., Nordin, J.D., Danila, R., 2004b. surveillance for influenzalike illness i tory care network. *Emerging Infectious L* 1806–1811.

Mollié, A., 1996. Bayesian mapping of diseas S., Richardson, S. (Eds.), *Markov Chain Mɪ Practice*, pp. 359–379. Chapman and Hall, ɪ

Monmonier, M., De Blij, H., 1996. *How to L* University of Chicago Press, Chicago.

Moore, D., 1999. Spatial diffusion of racco Pennsylvania, USA. *Preventive Veterinarʏ* 19–32.

Moran, P.A.P., 1948. The interpretation maps. *Journal of the Royal Statistical Sociɛ* 243–251.

Moran, P.A.P., 1950. Notes on continuous ; nomena. *Biometrika* **37**, 17–23.

Morris, S.E., Wakefield, J.C., 2000. Assessɪ risk in relation to a pre-specified sou P., Wakefield, J.C., Best, N.G., Brigs, D *Epidemiology*, pp. 153–184. Oxford U Oxford.

Morris, R.S., Wilesmith, J.W., Stern, M.V Stevenson, M.A., 2001. Predictive spaɪ alternative control strategies for the disease epidemic in Great Britain, 20 *Record* **149**, 137–144.

Morton-Jones, T., Diggle, P., Elliott, P., ɪ of excess environmental risk around Stone's test with covariate adjustɪ *Medicine* **18**, 189–197.

Muirhead, C., Darby, S., 1989. Royal meeting: Cancer near nuclear insta *the Royal Statistical Society Series A* ɪ

Müller, I., Betuela, I., Hide, R., 2002. of birthweights in Papua New Gɪ diet, environment and socio-econ of Human Biology **29**, 74–78.

Piantadosi, S., Byar, D., Green, S., 1988. The ecological fallacy. *American Journal of Epidemiology* **127**, 893–904.

Picardo, A., Guitian, F.J., Pfeiffer, D.U. 2007. Space-time interaction as an indicator of local spread during the 2001 FMD outbreak in the UK. *Preventive Veterinary Medicine* **79**, 3–19.

Pickle, L., Mungiole, M., Jones, G., White, A., 1996. *Atlas of United States Mortality*. National Center for Health Statistics, Hyattsville.

Plummer, M., Clayton, D., 1996. Estimation of population exposure in ecological studies. *Journal of the Royal Statistical Society Series B* **58**, 113–126.

Porphyre, T., McKenzie, J., Stevenson, M. 2007. A descriptive spatial analysis of bovine tuberculosis in intensively controlled cattle farms in New Zealand. *Veterinary Research* **38**, 465–479.

Price, J.C., 1984. Land surface temperature measurement for the split window channels of the NOAA 7 Advanced Very High Resolution Radiometer. *Journal of Geophysical Research* **8**, 7231–7237.

Pugliatti, M., Solinas, G., Sotgiu, S., Castiglia, P., Rosati, G., 2002. Multiple sclerosis distribution in Northern Sardinia – spatial cluster analysis of prevalence. *Neurology* **58**, 277–282.

R Development Core Team, 2006. *R: A Language and Environment for Statistical Computing*. R Foundation for Statistical Computing, Vienna.

Raso, G., Matthys, B., N'Goran, E., Tanner, M., Vounatsou, P., Utzinger, J., 2005. Spatial risk prediction and mapping of *Schistosoma mansoni* infections among schoolchildren living in western Cote d'Ivoire. *Parasitology* **131**, 97–108.

Raso, G., Vounatsou, P., Singe, B., N'Goran, E., Tanner, M., Utzinger, J., 2006a. An integrated approach for risk profiling and spatial prediction of *Schistosoma mansoni* – hookworm coinfection. *Proceedings of the National Academy of Sciences of the United States of America* **103**, 6934–6939.

Raso, G., Vounatsou, P., Gosoniu, L., Tanner, M., N'Goran, E., Utzinger, J., 2006b. Risk factors and spatial patterns of hookworm infection among schoolchildren in a rural area of western Côte d'Ivoire. *International Journal for Parasitology* **36**, 201–210.

Recuenco, S., Eidson, M., Kulldorff, M., Johnson, G., Cherry, B., 2007. Spatial and temporal patterns of enzootic raccoon rabies adjusted for multiple covariates. *International Journal of Health Geographics* **6**, 14.

Rezaeian, M., Dunn, G., St Leger, S., Appleby, L., 2004. The production and interpretation of disease maps: A methodological case-study. *The International Journal for Research in Social and Genetic Epidemiology and Mental Health Services* **39**, 947–954.

Ribeiro Jr, P., Diggle, P., 2001. geoR: a package for geostatistical analysis. *R News* **1/2**, 15–18.

Richardson, S., Monfort, C., 2000. Ecological correlation studies. In: Elliott, P., Wakefield, J., Best, N., Briggs, D. (Eds.), *Spatial Epidemiology Methods and Applications*, pp. 205–220. Oxford University Press, Oxford.

Ripley, B.D., 1976. The second-order analysis of stationary point processes. *Journal of Applied Probability* **13**, 255–266.

Ripley, B.D., 1977. Modelling spatial patterns *(with discussion)*. *Journal of the Royal Statistical Society Series B* **39**, 172–212.

Ripley, B., 1981. *Spatial Statistics*. John Wiley and Sons Ltd, Chichester.

Ripley, B., 1988. *Statistical Inference for Spatial Processes*. Cambridge University Press, Cambridge.

Robinson, T.P., 2000. Spatial analysis and geographic information systems in epidemiology and public health. *Advances in Parasitology* **47**, 81–128.

Robinson, T.P., Harris, R.S., Hopkins, J.S., Williams, B.G., 2002. Decision support for trypanosomiasis control: an example using a geographical information system in eastern Zambia. *International Journal of Geographical Information Science* **16**, 345–360.

Robinson, T.P., Franceschini, G., Wint, G.R.W. 2007. FAO's *Gridded Livestock of the World*. *Veterinaria Italiana* **43**.

Roche, L.M., Skinner, R., Weinstein, R.B., 2002. Use of a geographic information system to identify and characterize areas with high proportions of distant stage breast cancer. *Journal of Public Health Management Practice* **8**, 26–32.

Rogers, D.J., 2006. Models for vectors and vector-borne diseases. *Advances in Parasitology* **62**, 1–35.

Rogers, D.J., Hay, S.I., Packer, M.J., 1996. Predicting the distribution of tsetse flies in West Africa using temporal Fourier processed meteorological satellite data. *Annals of Tropical Medicine and Parasitology* **90**, 225–241.

Rogerson, P.A., 1997. Surveillance systems for monitoring the development of spatial patterns. *Statistics in Medicine* **16**, 2081–2093.

Rogerson, P.A., 2006. Statistical methods for the detection of spatial clustering in case-control data. *Statistics in Medicine* **25**, 811–823.

Rothenberg, R.B., Thacker, S.B., 1992. Guidelines for the investigation of clusters of adverse health events. In: Elliott, P., Cuzick, J., English, D., Stern, R. (Eds.), *Geographical and Environmental Epidemiology: Methods for Small-Area Studies*, pp. 264–277. Oxford University Press, Oxford.

Rothenberg, R.B., Steinberg, K.K., Thacker, S.B. (Eds.), 1990. National conference on clustering of health events. *American Journal of Epidemiology* **132**, S1–S202.

Rothman, K.J., 1990. A sobering start for the cluster busters' conference. *American Journal of Epidemiology* **132**, S6–S13.

Rowlingson, B., Diggle, P., (1993) Splancs: spatial point pattern analysis code in S-Plus. *Computers and Geosciences* **19**, 627–655.

Saaty, 1980. *The Analytic Hierarchy Process*. McGraw-Hill, New York.

Sabel, C., Gatrell, A., Löytönen, M., Maasiltad, P., Jokelainen, M., 2000. Modelling exposure opportunities: estimating relative risk for motor neurone disease in Finland. *Social Science and Medicine* **50**, 1121–1137.

Sadiq, R., Rodriguez, M.J., 2005. Interpreting drinking water quality in the distribution system using Dempster-Shafer theory of evidence. *Chemosphere* **59**, 177–188.

Sankoh, O.A., Yé, Y., Sauerborn, R., Müller, O., Becher, H., 2001. Clusters of childhood mortality in rural Burkina Faso. *International Journal of Epidemiology* **30**, 485–492.

Sanson, R.L., Pfeiffer, D.U., Morris, R.S., 1991. Geographic information systems: Their application in animal disease control. *Revue Scientifique et Technique de l'Office International des Epizooties* **10**, 179–195.

Sauders, B.D., Fortes, E.D., Morse, D.L., Dumas, N., Kiehlbauch, J.A., Schukken, Y., Hibbs, J.R., Wiedmann, M., 2003. Molecular subtyping to detect human listeriosis clusters. *Emerging Infectious Diseases* **9**, 672–680.

Savill, N.J., Shaw, D.J., Deardon, R., Tildesley, M.J., Keeling, M.J., Woolhouse, M.E., Brooks, S.P., Grenfell, B.T., 2006. Topographic determinants of foot and mouth disease transmission in the UK 2001 epidemic. *BMC Veterinary Research* **2**, 3.

Schabenberger, O., Gotway, C.A., 2005. *Statistical Methods for Spatial Data Analysis*. Chapman & Hall/CRC Press, Boca Raton.

Schlattmann, P., 1996a. The computer package DismapWin. *Statistics in Medicine* **15**, 931.

Schlattmann, P., 1996b. Covariate adjusted mixture models and disease mapping with the program DismapWin. *Statistics in Medicine* **15**, 919–929.

Schlesselman, J., 1982. *Case-Control Studies: Design, Conduct, Analysis*. Oxford University Press, New York.

Schober, E., Rami, B., Waldhor, T., Karimian-Teherani, D., 2001. Regional distribution of childhood onset diabetes mellitus in Austria–analysis of national registration from 1989 to 1999. *Wiener Klinische Wochenschrift* **113**, 491–495.

Schulman, J., Selvin, S., Merrill, D., 1988. Density equalized map projections: A method for analysing clustering around a fixed point. *Statistics in Medicine* **7**, 491–505.

Schwermer, H., Forster, K., Brülisauer, F., Chaubert, C., Heim, D., 2007. BSE, feed and cattle in Switzerland: Is there a spatial relation? *Veterinary Research* **38**, 409–418.

Scott, D.W., 1992. *Multivariate Density Estimation: Theory, Practice and Visualisation*. John Wiley & Sons, New York.

Selvin, S., Merrill, D.W., Erdmann, C., White, M., Ragland, K., 1998. Breast cancer detection: Maps of 2 San Francisco bay area counties. *American Journal of Public Health* **88** 1186–1192.

Sheehan, T.J., De Chello, 2005. A space-time analysis of the proportion of late stage breast cancer in Massachusetts, 1988 to 1997. *International Journal of Health Geographics* **4**, 15.

Sheehan, T.J., Gershman, S.T., MacDougall, L.A., Danley, R.A., Mroszczyk, M., Sorenson, A.M., Kulldorff, M., 2000. Geographic assessment of breast cancer screening by towns, zip codes, and census tracts. *Journal of Public Health Management Practice* **6**, 48–57.

Sheridan, H.A., McGrath, G., White, P., Fallon, R., Shoukri, M.M., Martin, S.W., 2005. A temporal-spatial analysis of bovine spongiform encephalopathy in Irish cattle herds, from 1996 to 2000. *The Canadian Journal of Veterinary Research* **69**, 19–25.

Smith, S.J. (Ed.), 1996. Centres for Disease Control (CDC) Symposium. Small area statistics in public health: Design, analysis, geographic and spatial methods. *Statistics in Medicine* **15**, 1827–1986.

Smith, K.L., DeVos, V., Bryden, H., Price, L.B., Hugh-Jones, M.E., Keim, P., 2000. *Bacillus anthracis* diversity in Kruger National Park. *Journal of Clinical Microbiology* **38**, 3780–3784.

Snijders, T., Bosker, R., 1999. *Multilevel Analysis: An Introduction to Basic and Advanced Multilevel Modelling*. Sage, London.

Snow, J., 1855. *On the Mode of Communication of Cholera*. John Churchill, London.

Snow, R.W., Gouws, E., Omumbo, J., Rapuoda, B., Craig, M.H., Tanser, F.C., Sueur, D.L., Ouma, J., 1998. Models to predict the intensity of *Plasmodium falciparum* transmission: applications to the burden of disease in Kenya. *Transactions* **92**, 601–606.

Snow, R.W., Craig, M.H., Deichmann, U., Sueur, D.L., 1999. A preliminary continental risk map for malaria mortality among African children. *Parasitology Today* **15**, 99–104.

Snyder, J.P., 1987. *Map Projections: A Working Manual*. United States Government Printing Office, Washington DC.

Song, C., Kulldorff, M., 2003. Power evaluation of disease clustering tests. *International Journal of Health Geographics* **2**, 9.

Song, C., Kulldorff, M., 2005. Tango's maximized excess events test with different weights. *International Journal of Health Geographics* **4**, 32.

Spiegelhalter, D., Abrams, K., Myles, J., 2002. *Bayesian Approaches to Clinical Trials and Health-Care Evaluation*. John Wiley and Sons, Chichester.

Spiegelhalter, D., Thomas, A., Best, N., Lunn, D., 2003. *WinBUGS User Manual–Version 1.4*. MRC Biostatistics Unit, Cambridge.

Spratt, B.G., 1999. *Independent Review of the Possible Health Hazards of the Large-scale Release of Bacteria during the Dorset Defence Trials*, p. 38. Ministry of Defence, London.

Stein, C.E., 2001. The cluster that never was: Germ warfare experiments and health authority reality in Dorset. *Journal of the Royal Statistical Society Series A* **164**, 23–27.

Stevenson, M.A., Wilesmith, J.W., Ryan, J.B., Morris, R.S., Lawson, A.B., Pfeiffer, D.U., Lin, D., 2000. Descriptive spatial analysis of the epidemic of bovine spongiform encephalopathy in Great Britain to June 1997. *Veterinary Record* **147**, 379–384.

Stevenson, M., Morris, R., Lawson, A., Wilesmith, J., Ryan, J., Jackson, R., 2005. Area-level risks for BSE in British cattle before and after the July 1988 meat and bone meal feed ban. *Preventive Veterinary Medicine* **69**, 129–144.

Stolley, P.D., Lasky, T., 1995. *Investigating Disease Patterns – The Science of Epidemiology*. Scientific American Library, New York.

Stone, R.A., 1988. Investigations of excess environmental risks around putative sources: Statistical problems and a proposed test. *Statistics in Medicine* **7**, 679–660.

Stoyan, D., Kendall, W.S., Mecke, J. 1995. *Stochastic Geometry and Its Applications*. John Wiley & Sons, Chichester.

Swain, P.H., 1978. Remote sensing: the quantitative approach. In *Remote Sensing: The Quantitative Approach*, P.H. Swain and S.M. Davis, (Eds.), pp. 136–187 & 221–223. McGraw-Hill, London.

Swayne, D., Cook, D., Buja, A., 1998. XGobi: Interactive Dynamic Data Visualization in the X Window System. *Journal of Computational and Graphical Statistics* **7**, 113–130.

Symanzik, J., Kötter, T., Schmelzer, S., Klinke, S., Cook, D., Swayne, D., 1998. Spatial Data Analysis in the Dynamically Linked ArcView/XGobi/XploRe Environment. *Computing Science and Statistics* **29**, 561–569.

Talbot, T.O., Kulldorff, M., Forand, S.P., Haley, V.B., 2000. Evaluation of spatial filters to create smoothed maps of health data. *Statistics in Medicine* **19**, 2399–2408.

Tango, T., 1995. A class of tests for detecting 'general' and 'focused' clustering of rare diseases. *Statistics in Medicine* **14**, 2323–2334.

Tango, T., 2000. A test for spatial disease clustering adjusted for multiple testing. *Statistics in Medicine* **19**, 191–204.

Tango, T., Takahashi, K., 2005. A flexibly shaped spatial scan statistic for detecting clusters. *International Journal of Health Geographics* **4**, 11.

Tatsuoka, M.M., 1971. *Multivariate Analysis: Techniques for Educational and Psychological Research*. John Wiley & Sons, New York.

Thomas, D.C., 1985. The problem of multiple inference in identifying point-source environmental hazards. *Environmental Health Perspectives* **62**, 407–414.

Thulke, H., Tischendorf, L., Staubach, C., Selhorst, T., Jeltsch, F., Muller, T., Schluter, H., Wissel, C., 2000. The spatio-temporal dynamics of a post-vaccination resurgence of rabies in foxes and emergency vaccination planning. *Preventive Veterinary Medicine* **47**, 1–21.

Tinline, R., Rosatte, R., MacInnes, C., 2002. Estimating the incubation period of racoon rabies: A time-space clustering approach. *Preventive Veterinary Medicine* **56**, 89–103.

Toledano, M., Jarup, L., Best, N., Wakefield, J., Elliott, P., 2001. Spatial variation and temporal trends of testicular cancer in Great Britain. *British Journal of Cancer* **84**, 1482–1487.

Tsutakawa, R., 1988. A mixed model for analyzing geographic variability in mortality rates. *Journal of the American Statistical Association* **83**, 37–42.

Tucker, C.J., Sellers, P.J. 1986. Satellite remote sensing of primary production. *International Journal of Remote Sensing* **7**, 1395–1416.

Turnbull, B.W., Iwano, E.J., Burnett, W.S., Howe, H.L., Clark, L.C., 1990. Monitoring for clusters of disease: Applications to leuke mia incidence in upstate New York. *American Journal of Epidemiology* **132**, S136–S143.

Upton, G.J.G., Fingleton, B., 1985. *Spatial Data Analysis by Example. Vol. 1. Point Pattern and Quantitative Data*. John Wiley & Sons, New York.

Upton, G.J.G., Fingleton, B., 1989. *Spatial Data Analysis by Example. Vol. 2. Categorical and Directional Data*. John Wiley & Sons, New York.

Urquhart, J., 1992. Studies of disease clustering: Problems of interpretation. In: Elliott, P., Cuzick, J., English, D., Stern, R. (Eds.), *Geographical and Environmental Epidemiology: Methods for Small-Area Studies*, pp. 278–285. Oxford University Press, Oxford.

Valencia, L.I., Fortes, B.P., Medronho, R.A., 2005. Spatial ascariasis risk estimation using socioeconomic variables. *International Journal of Environmental Health Research* **15**, 411–424.

Viel, J., Pobel, D., Carré, A., 1995. Incidence of leukaemia in young people around the La Hague nuclear waste reprocessing plant: A sensitivity analysis. *Statistics in Medicine* **14**, 2459–2472.

Viel, J.-F., Arveux, P., Baverel, J., Cahn, J.-Y., 2000. Soft-tissue sarcoma and non-Hodgkin's lymphoma clusters around a municipal solid waste incinerator with high dioxin emission levels. *American Journal of Epidemiology* **152**, 13–19.

Vinten-Johansen, P., Brody, H., Paneth, N., Rachman, S., Rip, M., 2003. *Cholera, Chloroform, and the Science of Medicine.* Oxford University Press, Oxford.

Vlachonikolis, I., Aletra, T., Georgoulias, V., 2002. Incidence of breast cancer on Crete, 1994–1995. *European Journal of Cancer* **38**, 574–577.

Wakefield, J.C., Kelsall, J.E., Morris, S.E., 2000. Clustering, cluster detection and spatial variation in risk. In: Elliott, P., Wakefield, J.C., Best, N.G., Briggs, D.J. (Eds.), *Spatial Epidemiology – Methods and Applications.* pp. 128–152. Oxford University Press, Oxford.

Wakefield, J., Quinn, M., Raab, G. (Eds.), 2001. Royal Statistical Society Meeting: Analysis and interpetation of disease clusters and ecological studies. *Journal of the Royal Statistical Society Series A* **164**, 1–303.

Waller, L. (1996) Statistical power and design of focused clustering studies. *Statistics in Medicine* **15**, 765–782.

Waller, L.A., Gotway, C.A., 2004. *Applied Spatial Statistics for Public Health Data.* John Wiley & Sons, New Jersey.

Waller, L., Lawson, A., 1995. The power of focused tests to detect disease clustering. *Statistics in Medicine* **14**, 2291–2308.

Waller, L.A., Turnbull, B.W., 1993. The effects of scale on tests for disease clustering. *Statistics in Medicine* **12**, 1869–1884.

Waller, L.A., Turnbull, B.W., Clark, L.C., Nasca, P., 1992. Chronic disease surveillance and testing of clustering of disease and exposure: Application to leukemia incidence and TCE-contaminated dumpsites in upstate New York. *Environmetrics* **3**, 281–300.

Waller, L., Carlin, B., Xia, H., Gelfand, A., 1997. Hierarchical spatio-temporal mapping of disease rates. *Journal of the American Statistical Association* **92**, 607–617.

Walsh, S.J., DeChello, L.M., 2001. Geographical variation in mortality from systemic lupus erythematosus in the United States. *Lupus* **10**, 637–646.

Walsh, S.J., Fenster, J.R., 1997. Geographical clustering of mortality from systemic sclerosis in the Southeastern United States, 1981-90. *The Journal of Rheumatology* **24**, 2348–2352.

Walter, S.D., 1992. The analysis of regional patterns in health data .2. The power to detect environmental effects. *American Journal of Epidemiology* **136**, 742–759.

Walter, S.D., 1993. Assessing spatial patterns in disease rates. *Statistics in Medicine* **12**, 1885–1894.

Walter, S., Martin Taylor, S., Marrett, L., 1999. An analysis of determinants of regional variation in cancer incidence: Ontario, Canada. In: Lawson, A., Biggeri, A., Böhning, D., Lesaffre, E., Viel, J.-F., Bertollini, R. (Eds.), *Disease Mapping and Risk Assessment for Public Health,* pp. 365–381. John Wiley and Sons Ltd, Chichester.

Wand, M.P., Jones, M.C., 1995. *Kernel Smoothing.* Chapman & Hall/CRC Press, Boca Raton, Florida.

Ward, M.P., 2001. Blowfly strike in sheep flocks as an example of the use of a time-space scan statistic to control confounding. *Preventive Veterinary Medicine* **49**, 61–69.

Ward, M.P., 2002. Clustering of reported cases of leptospirosis among dogs in the United States and Canada. *Preventive Veterinary Medicine* **56**, 215–226.

Ward, M.P., Carpenter, T.E., 1995. Infection of cattle in Queensland with bluetongue viruses. II. Distribution of antibodies. *Australian Veterinary Journal* **74**, 128–131.

Ward, M.P., Carpenter, T.E., 2000. Analysis of time-space clustering in veterinary epidemiology. *Preventive Veterinary Medicine* **43**, 225–237.

Wartenberg, D., 2001. Investigating disease clusters: Why, when and how? *Journal of the Royal Statistical Society Series A* **164**, 13–22.

Wartenberg, D., Greenberg, M., 1990. Detecting disease clusters: The importance of statistical power. *American Journal of Epidemiology* **132**, S156–S166.

Wartenberg, D., Greenberg, M., 1993. Solving the cluster puzzle: Clues to follow and pitfalls to avoid. *Statistics in Medicine* **12**, 1763–1770.

Webb, C.R., 2005. Farm animal networks: unravelling the contact structure of the British sheep population. *Preventive Veterinary Medicine* **68**, 3–17.

Webster, R., Oliver, M.A., Muir, K.R., Mann, J.R., 1994. Kriging the local risk of a rare disease from a register of diagnoses. *Geographical Analysis* **26**, 168–185.

Wilesmith, J., Stevenson, M., King, C., Morris, R., 2003. Spatio-temporal epidemiology of foot-and-mouth disease in two counties of Great Britain in 2001. *Preventive Veterinary Medicine* **61**, 157–170.

Williams, E.H., Smith, P.G., Day, N.E., Geser, A., Ellice, J., Tukei, P., 1978. Space-time clustering of Burkitt's lymphoma in the West Nile District of Uganda, 1961-1975. *British Journal of Cancer* **37**, 109–122.

Wint, G.R.W., Robinson, T.P., 2007. *Gridded Livestock of the World, 2007.* Food and Agriculture Organization of the United Nations, Animal Production and Health Division, Rome.

Wint, G., Robinson, T., Bourn, D., Durr, P., Hay, S., Randolph, S., Rogers, D., 2002. Mapping bovine tuberculosis in Great Britain using environmental data. *Trends in Microbiology* **10**, 441– 444.

Wylie, J.L., Cabral, T., Jolly, A.M., 2005. Identification of networks of sexually transmitted infection: A molecular, geographic, and social network analysis. *Journal of Infectious Diseases* **191**, 899–906.

Xia, H., Carlin, B., Waller, L., 1997. Hierarchical models for mapping Ohio lung cancer rates. *Environmetrics* **8**, 107–120.

Yang, G.-J., Vounatsou, P., Zhou, X.-N., Tanner, M., Utzinger, J., 2005. A Bayesian-based approach for spatio-temporal modeling of county level prevalence of *Schistosoma japonicum* infection in Jiangsu province, China. *International Journal for Parasitology* **35**, 155–162.

Zeiler, M., 1999. *Modeling Our World; The ESRI Guide to Geodatabase Design*. Environmental Systems Research Institute, Redlands, California.

Zheng, X., Pierce, G., Reid, D., Jolliffe, I., 2002. Does the North Atlantic current affect spatial distribution of whiting? Testing environmental hypotheses using statistical and GIS techniques. *ICES Journal of Marine Science* **59**, 239–253.

Index

Note: page numbers in *italics* refer to Figures and Tables.